From My
Heart
To Yours

Shaeah L♥ve

Edited by Coreen Boucher, www.lucentedits.com

Cover Image: On Wings of Light, by Atmara Rebecca Cloe

www.nwcreations.com

Photo of Shaeah by Marta Mora

www.martamoraphotography.ca

Please direct any comments, requests or questions to

connect@shaeahlove.com

www.shaeahlove.com

Produced by:

FriesenPress

Suite 300 – 852 Fort Street

Victoria, BC, Canada V8W 1H8

www.friesenpress.com

Distributed to the trade by The Ingram Book Company

Dedicated to all those I love, have loved and will ever love.
Love is the Force that Unites Us All

❤ Acknowledgments ❤

Special thanks to my mom who loves me unconditionally; my dad who challenges and adores me; my second mom who supports and encourages me; my brother, Jonah, who I adore; my sister, Suzannah, who inspires me; and my soul sister, Theda, who has always been there for me.

Also a very special thanks to all my mentors and teachers who believed in me especially when I didn't: Anjali, Anurag, Donna, Kealohi, Lawrence, Saraswati, Satyen, Stephen and Suzanne. Thank you to the accomplished ones who revealed more of the way: Ruth Ozeki and SARK.

Infinite gratitude and blessings to my editor, Coreen Boucher, who so gracefully and beautifully refined this book while maintaining its integrity and soul. I am grateful to everyone at FriesenPress for their care, service and support that has made publishing this book possible.

Deep heartfelt appreciation to all of my soul brothers and sisters who have walked some part of this path with me and who either shared their love with me, gave me an opportunity to share mine or both. And, of course, thank you to all who challenged me and gave me an opportunity to grow and learn more about myself, life and others.

Thank you to all my superheroes who have demonstrated and inspire a courageous, compassionate and heartfelt way of being; Blessed Teresa of Calcutta, Dalai Lama, Gandhi, Marianne Williamson and Nelson Mandela. Last, but not least, and most importantly is my Beloved, Majie, my match made in heaven, who enriches my life immensely. From the depths of my heart and soul I thank you for all of your incredible love and support.

♥ Contributors ♥

I have been incredibly blessed by all the support I have received from friends and family throughout the process of publishing this book. From the depths of my heart and the core of my soul, I thank you for believing in me and helping me to birth this book into being.

Albert, Marcy, Gabriella, Aviva & Jazlyn Fialkow	Ellie Willix	Mike Hermon
Alex Hutton	Erik Paulsson	Naomi & Nico teWinkel
Andrea Goldsmith	Erma Fialkow	Nina Clare Withrington
Andrew Rezmer	Farhana Dhalla	Patricia Murray
Andy Vine	Gary Wojciechowski	Penelope Bell
Anne Moyls	Gil Yaron	Prema Lee Gurreri
Ashish Raja	Heather Beck	Rachel & Louis Baxter Bourget
Ashley Hain	Heidi Michelle	Rachel Finer & Jeff Strong
Astraea Starr	Hils	Rodney Ost
Brenda & Sean Nixon	Ian Mackenzie	Romina Jones

Brenda, Wayne & Crystal Brennan	Joe Bundy	Rovena Skye
Callie & Jason Westlake	Johnathan Ikebuchi	Satyen & Suzanne Raja
Charles E Davis	Johnny Love	Sean Aiken
Chen Dror	Julia Larmour	Sobey Wing
Cheryl McClellan-Moody	Ki Michael Bouris	Sonny Davis
Chris Barbeau	Kris Palesch	Soorya & Jack Resels
Christina Godlewska	Lauren Kilbourn	Suzannah Fialkow
Christopher Fleck	Leigh Kankewitt	Sylvie Lalonde
Cindy Ferrige	Leslie Lewis	Tamarah Ney
Clint Carleton	Linda Robinson	Tanis Dagert
Coreen Boucher	Lisa Archibald	Terisa Adam
Craig & Joyce Clarke	Luca Emerald & Christian Prekratic	Theda Phoenix
Danielle Edmondson & Tim Ibbotson	Lynne Hilderman	Torsten
David H. Stewart	Majie Lavergne	Valeriana and Naeem
Denise Bertin-Maclean	Marc & Carrie Meyer	Veronica Silva
Diane Corbin	Marilyn Sheckter & Sam Fialkow	Vidan Gonthier
Donya and Gordon	Mark Kennedy	Wayne and Heather
Elinor Bazar	Melanie & Don McLove	Xilla

A Love Letter

Dearest You,

From the infinite depths of my heart, thank you. Thank you for taking your precious time to read and receive my offering. Thank you for letting me into your life and maybe even your heart. Thank you for delving into my world, heart and mind. Thank you for being on this wild and wonder-filled journey with me.

You matter. You make a difference. You've made a difference to me by simply opening up this book and letting me in. You are a unique and wonderous being that has a whole universe of amazingness to discover inside of you. I'm excited for you. Love, appreciate and enjoy yourself and your life as much as you can. It's a precious life. And you are a precious being.

We are perfectly imperfect, you and I, and loveable just as we are. In this way we are one and the same. Perfectly imperfect loveable precious beings.

I wish for you the most magical, beautiful, delightful, real and fulfilling life you can possibly live. I bless you on your journey however you choose to live it.

Infinite love & blissings,

Introduction

Who looks outside, dreams;
who looks inside, awakes.
~Carl Jung

Ultimately this is a love story. Would you expect anything less from someone who proclaims herself as Ms. Love? In this book I share the tools I have used for healing and transformation that have helped me to find the love and fulfillment I now have and that continues to grow and deepen. The most effective and powerful tool and the greatest form of love that I have discovered and live by is radical honesty both with myself and with others. That is why I have written this book in a style of free-flow with little or no editing. I intentionally don't hide anything or try to sound good. I have done my best to leave my writing in its original form as much as possible. I have taken out certain excerpts that seemed harmful to others or were completely superfluous.

This form of expression can be likened to improv. Improv theatre, dance and music is spontaneously created in the moment. This is a journey of breaking free, free of both external and self-imposed constraints and limitations. In the process of exposing myself as I am I have freed myself from shackles of fear, hatred and shame.

Radical honesty requires the willingness to dig deep into one's own heart and soul and along the way pass through the various layers and trappings of the mind. The mind is a tricky thing and will try to convince you of many things that aren't true.

At times, I think I am mentally ill. Does this thought sentence me to a life of misery? It could if I let it. I believe anyone who has any destructive, limiting or hurtful thoughts suffers from some degree of mental illness.

Luckily, we are not limited to or bound by our thoughts or experiences. We are beings of choice. Rick Hansen, the author of Buddha's Brain, said that we have two wolves in our heart, the wolf of hate and the wolf of love, and we can decide which wolf to feed. Science has now proven that our cells change and are affected by numerous factors including our thoughts and our environment. What we choose to focus on and what we surround ourselves with influences and shapes who we are and who we become.

Despite my lifelong struggle with unhealthy, unsupportive and destructive thinking, I have managed to live a full, rich and amazing life. I attribute this to my dedication to and faith in the power of love. Life has been difficult, at times unbearable. I've hidden my inner struggle from others, often suffering quietly and alone. Life may have been easier if I had come out a long time ago. Perhaps I could have received more help.

I've come to trust the natural unfolding of life and the belief that everything happens for a reason. My personal struggle with mental illness has forced me to dig deeper within myself for strength and to reach out to others for deeper connection and strength when I couldn't find it within myself.

The choice is ours. Do we continue to suffer quietly and feed the wolf of hate or do we share ourselves as we are and thereby release the shame and feed the wolf of love?

Writing this book was an ongoing practice of feeding the wolf of love. I explored and uncovered many parts of myself that had been long neglected or rejected and, in the process, became a more whole and integrated person. I continue to consciously choose to cultivate love as much as I can in every area of my life. Hence, the name Shaeah Love.

My given name is Shaeah Fialkow. I chose the name Shaeah Love as my radio personality when I started my radio show, Heart & Soul, in 2011 and it stuck. I've come to realize and experience that a name can hold certain power and influence. Taking on the last name Love offers a constant reminder and holds the energy and vibration of that which I seek to create and bring into the world. I am the love that I seek. This book is one of my boldest and most courageous expressions of my love, both for myself and for you.

Publishing this book is also one of the most terrifying things I have ever done. And believe me I have done many wild and daring things in my life. I have walked across hot coals in Japan, hitchhiked alone in Central America, dove in shark-infested waters at night, floated down the Nile in a felucca, bared my naked butt on stage in front of hundreds of people, and participated in shamanic journeys where I faced down my darkest demons.

The reason that publishing this book is so terrifying is because it is me baring my soul, revealing some of my deepest, darkest secrets. I fear that you will judge me and make decisions about who I am based on what I have written. So you may be wondering, why? Why do it? Believe me I have considered not doing it many times. I have sat on this book for months gathering the courage to publish it. Every time I think I've made the decision not to, something deep inside emerges compelling me to do so. It's about finding my voice, owning who I am and being a source of inspiration to others. It's about contributing and being of service. It's about courage, integrity and strength. It's about fulfilling my purpose. It's about truth and vulnerability. It's about being fully who I am and not hiding or pretending anymore. It's about freedom of expression, letting go and trusting that who I am and what I have to share is enough, is good and is of benefit to others. It's about being true to myself and about having faith. Ultimately it's about me loving myself just as I am. It's true, honest, heartfelt sharing. May it touch and inspire you. I offer this book as a ray of light and of hope. I offer it as my gift to you, from my heart to yours.

Enjoy the ride!

Please Note: This book has been edited as minimally as possible to maintain the integrity and soul of the writing. At places I have added commentary for clarification, which is distinguished by italics.

Prologue
A True Faery's Tale...

Once upon a time there was a shy young girl who often felt sad, lonely and in despair. She was extremely sensitive. She lived a lot of her life in fantasy to escape the pain and fear that she felt. She buried herself in books, television and movies. She loved faery tales and would often fantasize about being rescued by her own knight in shining armor. As she grew older, she would escape her life by travelling and acting, she could pretend to be other people, recreate herself with each new person she met and didn't have to face her own feelings. She visited many distant lands, met incredible people, had wild and wondrous adventures and yet—wherever she went, whatever she did—she couldn't escape the pain. At some point, the pain got so great that she even gave up on her dreams of being a great actress. She withdrew into herself and began to live a shallow existence and ultimately a lie.

No one knew of the true anguish she was experiencing, she hid it well and kept herself distracted and busy by trying to save the world. She became an environmental activist and a very involved community member. She owned a successful business, threw big amazing parties, was meeting people from all over the world and yet she was still unhappy, sad and lonely. She was even starting to become angry and didn't know why.

One day she met a handsome Knight, who did save her in a way, by opening the door for her to have a relationship with God. Shortly after, she met a great Shaman, who took both her and her Knight on a deep and long healing journey. She studied the Hawaiian Healing Arts with fervour and passion, hoping to finally fix and escape the pain that she felt. On this journey, she met a Divine Soul Sister with the most angelic voice, who would become one of her greatest allies

From My
Heart
To Yours

on the epic journey of her healing path. Even though she did experience immense love and joy through the healing spirit of Aloha, the pain continued to grow, and she couldn't escape the feeling that something was still missing. Something was calling her home …

At a great gathering of Wise Women, she participated in a shamanic journey, where her spirit guide, the moose, told her it was time to return to her birthplace. She left her Knight and her community to venture across the majestic Rockies and settled in the comfortable and cozy cave of her parents' basement. During this time, she reconnected with her blood family, looked after her young siblings and helped nurse her ailing grandmother back to health. And yet, she still was not happy, something was missing …

One evening she had an enchanting dance with a playful loving Fool who took her to meet a great Wizard and true WarriorSage. The Wizard promised to reveal to her the deep mysteries of life and help her return home to her true essence and to the great Source. This was an offer she couldn't refuse, no matter what the price! Sure enough, he was right. She had a great awakening and connected deeply with her true Self. She was so ecstatic and grateful that she vowed to dedicate her life to help others do the same, and she pledged her faithful allegiance to the great Wizard and the Path of the WarriorSage. However, this was not 'the fix' that she had hoped for. When she returned home, life was still the same and the unhappiness began to slowly seep in again. Luckily, her vow helped to guide her and to keep her committed to walking this new Path. The great Wizard and his Allies saw something special in her and believed in her even when she didn't. They offered her support and guidance to continue to walk the challenging and rewarding path of Truth, Freedom and Love.

This path was not an easy one. She encountered many outer and inner demons and walked through many dark nights of her soul. Some nights she barely made it out alive. At times she faltered and lost her way, but somehow she always managed to get herself back on the path (often with a little or a lot of help). It was during this time that her Angelic Soul Sister opened the door to the Realm of Possibility. Through the guidance of many great Teachers, she began to free herself from self-imposed limitations and to cultivate the skills for creating her own life. Life was still not perfect, and the way proved difficult; she stumbled and fell often. Miraculously, each time she picked herself up and continued to walk the path, she grew stronger and more alive.

One day, the great Wizard decided she was ready for a new level of initiation into self-mastery and introduced her to his teacher, the Grand Master. This began a wild and fascinating journey into the workings of her mind. In her exploration, she began to discover that all of her suffering originated in her mind, she learned that she had created her own prison and—quite astonishingly—that she held the key. Even though a part of her still wanted to blame all the trolls and bad guys, she realized that the more responsibility she took for her own life and her own happiness, the more freedom and choice she had. As she began to awaken to this new level of freedom and choice, she started to look at the things that brought her the greatest joy and made them a priority in her life. She began her mornings with dancing or yoga; she took regular walks in nature; she joined a choir so she could sing her heart out; she began to Shimmy for her Soul (belly dancing); she spent more quality time with her family and friends. She grew stronger, healthier and more vital each day.

One morning, she realized how strong and vital she felt from her yoga practice and decided she wanted to share the benefits of yoga with others. She mentioned this to the Grand Master, and he told her about the Supreme Guru of Compassion, Kripalu. She was so touched and inspired by Kripalu's message of love and compassion that she went to live at his center in the Berkshire Hills to immerse herself in the study of yoga and to receive Kripalu's blessing to share yoga with the world. At the end of her time at the Kripalu Center, while kayaking amongst the lotus flowers, she received the message that it was now time to return to the magical faery land of Mt. Elphinstone.

With the loving support of her family and community, she made the big journey back 'home.' She would take long walks along the beach or in the forest, dance with her faery friends, teach yoga, write, offer guidance and support others to heal and grow. She now lives happily, with immense gratitude and reality, in a magical faery forest by the sea, where she shares her inspiration, wisdom and gifts with whoever is ready and willing to receive them. Psyche! Of course that couldn't last long. She was happy and content for a while but something was still missing ... she was still alone.

From My
Heart
To Yours

One day while walking in the forest, she met a Prince who shared her passion for nature, dance, yoga and play. He invited her to live with him in his beautiful castle built on a hill overlooking the sea. She thought she had finally 'arrived' and could now live happily ever after. Little did she know, demons still lurked in the shadows of her subconscious. Doubt, insecurity, judgment, unworthiness and comparison started to poke their nasty heads into her hopes and dreams. The walls of the castle, which had once made her feel safe and secure, now loomed over her like a prison, heightening her feelings of isolation. The wicked witch of her psyche turned her Prince into a toad and once again she was alone. Misery overtook her, and she fell into a dark hole of confusion and despair. She was just about to fall down the rabbit hole when suddenly …

Her Father scooped her up in his loving arms and took her back to the family home to be cared for and supported. Her faery Godmother used her magic vibes to find a great metaphysical healer. He was known throughout the land for inventing a powerful machine that could magically heal people. After ten treatments of spinning in the magical machine and talking about love, she regained her strength and felt better enough to return to the land that meets the sea. She was welcomed home by a gathering of all her most treasured friends and family (except for her mom, who lived in a far-off land and was beamed in through the wonders of cyberspace). During this magnificent celebration of her life, she finally got how much she was loved and supported. With renewed strength and hope, she decided to finally put all the tools she had learned to use and began to create the life that she had always dreamed of.

She moved to a magical island, with pristine wilderness, a community of shared values and the home to the famous Hollyhock. It was here that she met many great teachers that generously shared their wisdom and knowledge. One of her greatest thrills was when she met one of her own personal heroes, the amazing SARK, who taught her about miracles, the marvelous messy middle and about how to manifest rainbows. She was deemed a Transformational Change Agent and took on the mission of boldly beaming and sharing her creatively blessed Self. With her newfound superpowers, she got the courage to start her own radio show, Heart & Soul, on which she gets to spread love through inspirational music and words.

One stormy evening at the Raven's den on the land of Hollyhock, she met a great Spiritual Master who opened the portal to the wonders of Loving Presence. She began to experience a whole new way of being in which she could rest more in the mystery and be grateful for what is. The nourishment of this work—mixed with the purity of the land, the water, the air and the hearts of the people who surrounded her—gave her an ever-growing sense of wholeness and well-being. She began to feel the most rested and at home she had ever felt. Could this be it? Would she finally be happy?

Winter came with a vengeance. Storm after storm blew in. The days grew shorter and darker. Her aches and pains got stronger as the days grew colder and damper. Despite the long walks in the woods to keep her blood pumping and her energy flowing and despite the many gatherings by the fire that kept her heart warm with the company of her friends, her body and heart continued to ache and her mind remained restless and uneasy.

Each night she would return to a cold and empty bed and had no one to keep her warm in those long cold nights, except for her pet lion. One day she received a call for help from her dear Mom, who needed her to stoke the home fires while she took a long overdue vacation to warmer lands. She grabbed her parka and embarked on a journey to the Great White North, otherwise known as the Peace Country. A fitting place to go in the search for inner peace. A thick blanket of snow covered the land, all was indeed still and peaceful. Many miles from any civilization, she took this opportunity to go into a deep silent meditation in search of her own inner peace and harmony. For five grueling days, she battled the demons of her mind and withstood armies of sensation and thoughts. Seduced by all manner of temptation, she held strong and steady to her course and emerged a changed woman. And this is where our tale begins …

And the day came when the risk to remain tight in a bud was more painful than the risk it took to blossom.
~ Anais Nin

FEBRUARY 21, 2012
PEACE COUNTRY, ALBERTA

So I'm finally making the commitment to write. At least a little bit every day and see what comes from it. Part of me has high expectations of something brilliant and another part of me fears utter failure or, at the very best, drivel. But hey, it's the effort that matters, no attachments to the outcome, right?! Just finally listening to and fulfilling the ever nagging voice to write. Write what? So many grand ideas. The latest I had this morning was something I can't even remember. It's so hilarious how every idea I get seems like it's going to be the next best seller, and yet I don't even get a dozen words out about it. Well, that's all going to change. I'm starting out with a 30-minute commitment a day and then we'll see how it goes and take it from there.

It's been an interesting time. At times it feels like a midlife crisis, and yet it feels like I've been in that for the last eight years or so. The elusive search for the self, for meaning, for purpose, for happiness, for fulfillment. I just completed 5 days of Vipassana at my mom's on my own.

VIPPASSANA

Vipassana which means to see things as they really are, is one of India's most ancient techniques of meditation. In the Buddhist tradition, it means insight into the true nature of reality. It was taught in India more than 2500 years ago as a universal remedy for universal ills. Said to have been the teaching of Buddha, it is meant to

cultivate mindfulness and a state of equanimity.[1]

The first and only time I took a 10-day Vipassana Meditation retreat was in 2002 just after I did my first Lomi Lomi (Hawaiian Shamanic Arts) Training. I remember it being quite challenging. I had to create a nest of pillows around me to be able to sit for any length of time and, even then, I experienced a significant amount of pain and restlessness of the mind. On day five, during one of my meditations, there was a moment when I experienced a flash of light in my body and mind and emerged from that sit without any pain and with a real life experience of true inner peace. Up until that point, inner peace was something I had just read about and was wary that it even existed. It exists alright! I was able to maintain that inner peace for some time but, as I emerged back into life and lost my meditation practice, the activity of the mind increased. I have since been able to touch into that sense of inner peace at certain times of quietude, when being in nature, moments or periods of contentment or in deep meditation. I have come to realize that a daily meditation practice is essential to my well-being, and I have a commitment to meditate at least once a day and am working towards ongoing mindfulness in everyday life.

I got the Vipassana schedule off the Internet and did it with a couple of revisions. Well, they had walking contemplation twice a day when I went, so I added that, and I shortened the 2-hour meditation to one and a half and sometimes 1 hour. And added one and a half hours of yoga. Plus I'm doing the Master Cleanse, so it's been a time of major purification. I experienced a lot of intense pain during my sits, sometimes unbearable. *I chose to do 'strong determination' meditation sits, which means staying completely still and simply observing the fluctuation of thought and sensation. This allows for the dissolution of deep dysfunctional patterns of the bodymind, our sankharas (mental formations—essentially either craving or aversion), which are said to be the root cause of emotional and physical pain.* I did my best to maintain a sense of calm, peace, equanimity, but it was really hard. I still don't like or understand pain and suffering. Although I'm beginning to suspect that it's a form of motivation to pursue something more, something deeper. Some say it guides us back to our soul.

I have gotten clearer that I want to be involved with helping people live a happy and fulfilling life. It sounds ridiculous saying that as I've been doing that most of my life, but I wasn't sure about it. Or the delivery of it didn't seem quite right, not quite me. I've been exploring this idea to work with youth and, all the while, it's been terrifying and intimidating me to the point where I haven't made any progress on it in years. I'm getting closer. I've talked to a couple of people about the possibilities, and I have an idea of what kind of program or course to offer them. It's about life, well-being and living a healthy happy life. Exploring that with youth, together. What that means, what that looks like, how to create it for themselves. It's exciting me actually. It has pushed me through my fear into enthusiasm. It's funny, the idea came to me on day four of my meditation and, of course, my mind went off on all these ideas about how it's going to become hugely successful, I'll get a reputation throughout the land and go on tours, all the schools will want my program, and how they'll create a movie about me. I am sooo hilarious. Always looking for that moment of fame and glory, even now.

Speaking of glory …I also got the idea of a one-woman show, again. *(I've had this idea before. I get a lot of ideas, as you'll come to know.)* But this time, even clearer and more exciting. I would really love to do it, whether I'll get the gumption for it is yet to be seen. I feel the next phase of my life is about the next level of my offering. My next truest, authentic expression. I'm still looking for that stroke of brilliance that will make it big, make ME big! Part of me thinks, "Why not? Why not go for brilliance, success, fortune?" Another part of me is wary of doing things for the wrong reason, from a place of ego rather than true heart and inspiration.

I have no idea what will become of me or what I'll do, but I do know that the most important aspect of this journey is to keep having faith in myself, keep honouring what's true and important to me, give generously with my whole heart and soul and do my best to enjoy the process along the way. What will be will be. Every time I think of that phrase, I flash back to a scene of me singing "Que Sera Sera" in a fringe play I was in, *Ding Dong the Bitch is Dead.* Hilarious. I played Dorothy. That was a fun role. I do love to perform. I need to honour that and keep allowing that part of myself to be expressed.

I have something to offer, something of value, I need to believe in that, know that and just keep offering. Sooner or later, I may make my fortune or not, but I'll at least be fulfilled in the effort. Have no regrets, right?! I am curious what will come, how, when, where, with whom? It's all a mystery. Steeped in the mystery, once again. I guess I'm starting to get a little more comfortable with the unknown. It comes back to that faith, trusting myself, trusting the grand plan, the Divine, God.

Trust and surrender, fascinating concepts/challenges, not sure what to call them. Ways of being, ultimately. I did have a breakthrough during my meditation about trust and surrender. Again on day four, I was doing surrender yoga, and I was getting frustrated and impatient, and finally I came to this point where I could see I had a choice to take control or let go, truly trust and surrender. It felt like a test, and a voice came back saying it was. And I'm glad and surprised to say that I passed. I lay there, I let go, didn't budge, trusted, surrendered and it felt good.

SURRENDER YOGA/MEDITATION
(Sahaja Yoga)

In Surrender Meditation, you don't use your will to guide your attention, control your body, or manage your energy. Instead you give over the entire process to the divine energies and let them do their work. Surrender Meditation begins with a prayer to God or whatever is divine to you. There can be many styles of this prayer, but the essence is that you pray that your meditation be blessed. Pray to give over your body, mind, emotions and life to God.

Sahaja Yoga is different from other yogas because it begins with Self-Realization.
~ Shri Mataji Nirmala Devi

Just a moment ago, I thought, "Wow, I could keep writing forever ..." then all of a sudden I became blank and had nothing more to say. Fascinating. My one major intention and commitment in my writing is to be as real, honest and transparent as possible.

People in transition are looking for support in saying yes to their own voice. Often, the systems we put in place to keep us secure are keeping us from our more creative selves.[2]
~ Patricia Ryan Madson

I want to live my life real, raw and authentically so why wouldn't my writing be the same, as it's an extension and expression of me. This will help me get clearer on who I am, and I'm hoping in the process to be a source of inspiration, help or at least amusement to others. It's interesting, this desire to benefit others, to be a source of help, good, something that people want or need. Is that just human nature, is it ego or is it necessary, like a glue that binds us together? Otherwise we might just take to being islands, on our own, isolated and separate. For some reason there is this driving force to connect, to share, to merge, to love. It always comes back to that for me—love.

I came to a point in my life, it was actually when I was in Israel a couple years back, when I was walking the streets of Jerusalem alone. There I was, walking these cobble stone streets filled with rich culture and history, and I thought, "This is empty and meaningless without someone to share it with." At that moment I became crystal clear that I wanted to share my life with somebody. Up until then, I had hints of doubt, of whether I wanted to give up my freedom. The ability to do what I wanted whenever I wanted, go wherever I wanted. But what's the point if I'm alone? Not for me; I'm a lover. I'm meant to share my life with someone. I have so much love to give, and yes, I know I can share my love with anyone and everyone. But an intimate partner kind of love is different. That's the journey I'd like to take and explore with a willing participant. My beloved. Where are you? Whenever shall we meet? That is the question and the next mystery to be solved in the great life of Shaeah. Time is up. I bid adieu until we meet again.

There is no turning back, we should concern ourselves only with the best way of going forward.
~ Paulo Coelho

Okay, I'm back. I couldn't stay away. Thirty minutes was the minimum, right? I have so much I want to share. So much that's racing around in my head, and I'm starting to quite enjoy this. I finally see this as a way to share all the things I've been wanting to but haven't had the chance, the opportunity, the moment, the courage. So many visions, fears, challenges, insights, hopes, dreams, stories. I've been waiting for so long, for that right time, right place, right inspiration, right conditions, right person. When—really—all I had to do was start. That's the key with all things, and I've known this, but sometimes it's easier said than done. Just start. I don't have to have it all figured out. I just need to start. This is exciting. This seems like a profound and powerful moment. A true breakthrough. I've been waiting for so long to do so many things and haven't. Have felt so stuck, afraid, immobilized, suppressed, blocked. So caught in fear, doubt, self-criticism, distraction. I often wonder where all the self-hate comes from, how I could be such a powerful force working against myself, my own worst enemy. But I guess it's my journey; there's something to be learned in it, to perhaps share with others. I've come a long way, Baby! ;-)

Yes, I'm going to use winks in my writing. I really like them. They're playful and fun. And that's how I want my writing to be, as well as deep and profound, of course. I want to be engaging, intriguing, compelling, spell binding, delightful, mysterious, enlightening, uplifting, inspiring, informative, creative, innovative, heartwarming, brilliant. I want to be all of that and so much more. I want you to like me. Actually, I want you to fall in love with me, adore me and, in the process of falling in love with me, I want you to fall in love with yourself. That brings a smile to my face. I know it may sound corny, but that's what's truly in my heart.

Yes, what's truly in my heart. That's what I want to share with you. The truest, deepest essence of my being. I want to be known, seen and appreciated. Isn't that okay? A part of it seems so true, good and real, and another part of it seems needy or egotistical. But I think it's in the intention behind it, don't you? The purity of it. And it's not purely selfish, for I also want that for you. I believe that's what we all want at the core. Maybe I'm deluded. Who cares? It's what's in my heart so I'm going with it. This is fun. I hope you appreciate and enjoy my ramblings.

I do care what you think. I know I probably shouldn't, but I do. I care what others think. I've tried so hard to not, but I do, so I may as well be honest about it. I had a teacher once who claimed he had broken free from that; he didn't care what anyone thought of him. I envied him. I could see his freedom in that. I aspired to that, I worked and strived really hard to get there, but I couldn't. And now I've realized it doesn't matter; the freedom comes from the acceptance of it, being honest about it and being who I am anyway. Not-so-secretly hoping that you'll like me. At least I no longer try to get you to like me. I've grown out of the trying. I think, I hope. I think I've gotten wise enough to know that people actually like me more if I'm real and honest about who I am; they'll definitely trust me more. That's for sure. I do like pretending, but I'll save that for the stage, for performing. But actually, having written that, I've realized that I like being authentic even more. Even in performing. I like presenting my truest self. That incredibly vulnerable, scary place that's so raw and enlivening. It's when I feel the most alive, when I'm in that exposed place. At times the self-critic still comes in and tells me all the ways that I could have been better and more brilliant, but—oh well. I'm working through that.

I have so many visions for how I want the world to be, but I'll save those for another time. This thought just came up so I thought I'd share it. I guess I'm floundering for what to say so I'll take that as my cue to bid adieu once again, my friend. Thanks for listening. And I hope it brings you as much pleasure and enjoyment reading it as it has brought me while writing it.

Okay, I'm actually on my lunch break, but I just had all these ideas that came flooding to me that I needed to share. I got the title of the book as I was sitting there sipping my maple syrup cayenne lemonade (notice that it has all the flavours covered: sweet, sour and spicy!)

observing the sea of thoughts floating through my head and thinking how great writing is, what a saving grace for all these thoughts that I constantly have and how addictive it could be. I was musing how sweet this morning's sharing was, sharing from my heart to yours, and that's it! That's when I got it, the title of the book, *From My Heart To Yours*! Isn't that great?! Perfect, really. So sweet and true.

And then, of course, my mind went into its grand imaginings of how big this book would become, how popular, a bestseller! ;-) Oh, so sweet. So fun. I decided that I'm going to just keep writing until I have 333 pages and call that my book. I wasn't even sure if that's a good length for a book, I just love that number. Threes have a special significance for me, I'm sure I'll get into that at some other point. Anyway, I went to the book that I am currently reading, *Yoga and the Quest for the True Self* by Stephen Cope (a brilliant book by the way, I highly recommend it), and it ends on page 341. How amazing is that?! *I intuited a good length for a book.* That's what I love about life—those sweet little magical synchronistic moments that let you know you're on the right track.

Sigh. I feel good being back on the path. I was feeling pretty lost there for a while. "Sometimes we have to lose ourselves to find ourselves again"; that phrase came to me from a voice in the middle of one of my moments of grace during my Vipassana sit. It was right after the same voice said to me, "Welcome home" and I said, "Thank God, I was feeling so lost." It's good to be home.

There are four questions of value in life, Don Octavio.
What is sacred? Of what is the spirit made?
What is worth living for and what is worth dying for?
The answer to each is the same. Only love.
~ Lord Byron

I just got back from my walk with tons of new things I want to share. My mind was swimming, actually flooding with ideas. I take a walk every day; it's one of my commitments to myself, among many others. I have slowly and consistently been making commitments to myself, to do the things that contribute to my well-being, that bring me joy, and that I absolutely love to do. I wonder if you have commitments to yourself, if you do the things that bring you joy on a regular basis or even if you know what those things are. If you don't, I wonder why. I strongly recommend finding out and making those things a priority. It will transform your experience of life. It did mine. It was actually out of necessity because I had gotten to a point where I wasn't enjoying life at all, so much so that I didn't want to live anymore. That's happened a few times. The point is that I had to take a good hard look at my life and get really clear on what's important to me and make my life about that so I had a life worth living. Now I do. I don't dread getting up in the morning anymore. That's a relief. The daily commitments I've made to myself are: walking, meditating, yoga, dance and music, and today I've added writing. I also have ongoing commitments of personal self-care, like baths, massages, eating healthy, thinking positively, continual learning, being honest, connecting with friends and family, communing with nature and having fun. I lead a pretty amazing life, but it was a long hard road to get here. And, even now, I face the ongoing challenges of self-doubt, laziness, fear, procrastination, self-sabotage, insecurity, and so on, but that's what keeps motivating me to dig deeper.

I'm trying to think of all the things I thought to share with you on my walk. It always sounds so brilliant in my head. I remember one thing very clearly; as I walked in the crisp clear air with the sun beaming on my head, I noticed that I am very excited and happy. Probably the most excited I've been in a long time. About this new venture, this journey of expressing myself authentically. It truly is a journey of discovery. I have no idea what's going to reveal itself and neither do you, so we're on this journey together—you and I—and it's exciting. It truly is an unfolding.

**The soul walks not upon a line, neither
does it grow like a reed. The soul unfolds itself,
like a lotus of countless petals.
~ Kahlil Gibran, *The Prophet***

I remembered one of the books I had an idea to write once, *Red Lotus Blossoming*, the story of my journey of awakening, so here it is.

This is my blossoming, and I do it for you. From my lotus heart to yours. There I go getting all corny again, but I love it. I know that writing this book won't always be this fun—or maybe it will. On my walk, I had flashes of days in the future where I could potentially curse this commitment to write and could have things going on that I dread to reveal to you and share. But we'll cross that bridge when and if we come to it. For now I'll hold the vision that the writing will all flow like warm sweet honey. Yum! Life is certainly a wild and wacky ride, never know what's around the next corner. Well, my friend, have to go and keep a commitment I've made to a dear friend of mine. But you guessed it … I'll be back! ;-)

Sooner than I thought. Interesting, talking about commitments, my friend hasn't seemed to have kept hers. That's an ongoing challenge for her, and I see how it affects her life. But I still love her; she's my deepest soul sister, Theda. Someone asked me once if I had anyone in my life who I felt totally accepted by and who loved me for who I am, who I could share anything with, and she's that person. Pretty much the only person at this point. Of course, I know my mom loves me unconditionally, but there are still some things I don't feel comfortable sharing with her. I think it's really important to have someone in your life you can totally be yourself with, ideally everyone, and especially your beloved, but I know it's not always the case. A lot of people feel they have to pretend or hide; I only say that because I did for most of my life. That part of me that wanted to be liked kept me wary of sharing certain things or presenting myself in ways that were appropriate or likeable.

That makes me think about my singing, and it makes me chuckle. Singing was one of the things I thought about on my walk. How much I love to sing and how bad I am at it. Well, not terrible. I know I have moments in which I even sound pretty good, but the problem is that's not consistently so. But I love singing so much that it hasn't stopped me. Well, not anymore. It did for the longest time.

In grade three, I had just moved to a new town and started going to a new school. They had a choir, and I was so thrilled to be in it. I think I was only in it for a few days or a week, at the most, when the teacher asked me to leave. I think that is one of the cruelest things anyone has ever done to me. I can't remember her reasoning, something about not having a good ear. I imagine it was because I was singing so loud due to my enthusiasm and excitement. As you can imagine, that scarred me for most of my life. I'm still working through some of the self-consciousness about singing, but mostly I don't let it stop me. It just brings me too much joy. I often had fantasies of becoming the lead singer of some great funk or rock or soul band. Honestly, I still do fantasize about being a great singer. I fantasize that someday I'll break through some block and—voila—this amazing voice will come through. Perhaps someday. Who knows, it could be possible.

I love living in the realm of possibility, something I picked up from Landmark. Why not believe that anything is possible? You'll get to know, if you haven't already guessed, that I'm quite the dreamer. I remember being quite shocked when a soul sister deemed me as a dreamer when she was deciding archetypes for all the women who worked together and for a tarot deck that we were going to create. But it's true, I am a dreamer. I like to think of myself more as a visionary. I do get lots of ideas and innovations but, most of the time, I'm so overwhelmed by it all that I become immobilized and do nothing. That's been one of my greatest challenges in life: wanting, seeing, imagining so much and doing so little. Truly, though, I have lived an extraordinary life. I was going through all the things that I've done when I was thinking of my write-up for the one-woman show I want to do. It went like this: Shaeah has lived more lives than a cat, having been an actor, stage manager, waitress, secretary, world traveller, English teacher, Taiko drummer, theatre manager, clown, singer, business owner, store manager, board member, circus performer, event producer, mind clearer, yoga teacher, massage instructor, enlightenment master, wizard trainer, filmmaker, financial advisor, property manager, tantrika, landscaper, dancer, healer, musician, visual artist, cook, environmental activist, consultant and spiritual guide, and now I can add writer! ;-) Yippee!! Quite the life, eh?! And I still have ambitions of so much more …bestselling author, movie star, Hollywood filmmaker, world leader and guest on the Oprah and David Letterman shows. Ending suffering on the planet, world peace, you know—the usual stuff. I feel my energy starting to drain a little, and I sense a niggling of doubt, a fear of you judging me. For thinking I'm futile or juvenile or too naïve, too idealistic.

Sometimes I truly do see how it's possible: world peace, that is, and the end of suffering. They showed part of it at the end of the movie, *Thrive*. Yes, it would take a lot, a major shift in consciousness, a lot of changes and sacrifices on behalf of some people, but come on people, for the greater good of all! Maybe that's some communism that I absorbed from my grandfather. I don't think he was really a communist. In fact, he defected from the Russian army after he liberated my grandmother from one of the concentration camps in Poland just before the fall of Hitler. Isn't that quite the story?

So, yes, I have deep roots of survival in me. But, honestly, doesn't everyone deep down want good for all beings? Isn't that our truest nature? We are all connected after all. Can't you feel the pain of the people suffering in the world? I can. I've learned to numb it, or at least manage it, mostly with yoga and meditation. But if I really open up, I feel it. It almost killed me once or, should I say, I almost killed myself because of it. It was when I was starting to wake up, doing Enlightenment/ Illumination Intensives, and one of my awakening moments was to the pain and suffering of all beings. It stayed with me for months, literally drove me crazy. I could barely get out of bed, I hurt too much. I would scream and wail for hours and days. I called a crisis line once, but they couldn't help me. *I don't remember why exactly they couldn't help. Upon reflection, I think it's because I was in a state where 'nothing would help.'* I was at a complete loss of what to do. I couldn't function. I couldn't get a job. I was doing massage from my house but, of course, I was barely getting any calls. I was in no condition to give sessions.

In desperation I went for a rebirthing session and out came so much anger at God. I cried, yelled and screamed at her/him for the entire session. I left the session feeling like a raw open wound. I didn't find the relief I'd been hoping for. That night I made myself a bath, got out my boyfriend's razor blades and tried to slit my wrists. I started to pierce the skin, but something wouldn't let me go through with it. I laid there crying and begging to let me do it or, if not, then tell me what I should live for. Suddenly, there it was—a voice—and it told me, "'Dance." The answer seemed strange and quite insignificant, but somehow it resonated with something deep within me. Live to dance. Dance is one of the most powerful ways I connect to Spirit, but I'd lost touch with it. Somehow, that gave me just enough of a glimmer to keep going. I had scars for a couple weeks, but nobody noticed. *I was living quite isolated at the time; the only person who saw me was my boyfriend, and we weren't connecting. I can be good at making myself invisible.* That was definitely one of my darkest times, but I've had others.

This is good, this is really good to talk about this stuff, quite therapeutic. I hope you don't think I'm making light of any of it. It was all very real and all necessary for some strange reason. I don't know if I've figured out exactly why, but that's where the faith comes in. I guess that's the thing I keep coming back to each time that I hit a challenging point in life. It calls forth a deeper faith in me. I have to trust that it's all for some greater good.

I feel the need to say something about the Enlightenment/ Illumination Intensive. Having reread this last excerpt, I can see how you might be left with the wrong idea about the process. It's not the Enlightenment/ Illumination Intensive that made me crazy or made me suicidal. I was already heading in that direction. I was already suffering. The Enlightenment/ Illumination Intensive speeds up the process of evolution and brings things to the surface that have been hidden, repressed and unconscious. I firmly believe that everything that has happened in my life has been a blessing in some way, made me a more compassionate, aware, loving and wise person. Enlightenment/ Illumination Intensives were a huge part of my life for many years are. At the first intensive that I participated in, I had a direct experience of who I am. It was one of the most liberating, empowering and life-affirming experiences of my life. Then and there, I chose to dedicate my life to supporting others to have that level of liberation. Being involved in Enlightenment/ Illumination Intensives gave meaning and purpose to my life and helped me to be a more real, honest, authentic, connected and fulfilled person. I recommend Enlightenment/ Illumination Intensives to anyone seeking liberation, connection and/or deeper understanding of yourself, life or others.

ENLIGHTENMENT / ILLUMINATION INTENSIVE

Enlightenment/ Illumination Intensive is a group retreat designed to enable a spiritual enlightenment experience within a relatively short time. Devised by Americans Charles and Ava Berner in the 1960s, the format combines the self-enquiry meditation method popularised by Ramana Maharshi with interpersonal communication processes, such as the dyad structure

You know, I have way more to say in my head than I do in real life, well, than I'm willing to say, I guess. It's just that I don't want to impose myself on others. It never seems like the right time; there's something more important to do or someone else has something to share. It really bothered me, those people who just natter on and who don't pay attention or seem to care whether anyone is interested in hearing what they are saying or not. That's the brilliant thing about this book, I can natter on about whatever, and you have the choice to keep reading, put the book down, throw it away, use it as a paperweight, give it away, or stay up all night glued to every word. Hee hee, you know which one I hope for, but really it doesn't matter. And I don't mean that I will take advantage of your listening and share mindlessly about ridiculous things—or maybe I will. I guess it's all perspective. But I do intend for my words to be meaningful and to touch you in some way. The question arises once again, why is that so important to me? Why this incessant need to influence, to have an effect, to connect? The answer once again, "Isn't that why we are here? Aren't we here to share and connect from the deepest most authentic place? Isn't that the true fulfillment of life?" Maybe not, maybe it's different for everyone. I can only truly speak for and from myself, so that's what I will happily continue to do. ;-)

I'll have you know that I am writing to you between intervals of dancing and staring up at the expansive twilit sky, just a tint of rose lingers at the horizon from the amazing Albertan sunset. The northwesterly wind that was blowing so fiercely earlier has subsided, stars just starting to sparkle. Peace is in the air. Candles are lit, I dance my prayer. This writing is now sacred. Wow, I just remembered that it is the new moon. So, yes indeed, this is sacred! What a perfect day to begin this book. If you didn't know, the new moon is a powerful time to set new intentions and to begin new projects so that the energy for it builds with the moon. I often host or participate in new moon circles, which are traditionally done with only women. Those times have been extremely powerful opportunities to connect, share,

From My

𝔥eart

To Yours

inspire, celebrate and simply just be with, enjoy and appreciate each other's presence.

NEW MOON CIRCLES

In ancient times, women in communities would gather together around the bleeding portion of their cycles, at the time of the new moon.

Modern circles are called Red Tent Temples, Moon Lodge gatherings and so forth. The purpose of the gathering is to honour women, reclaim the female sense of community in a small gathering, and to honour the cycles of life.[3]

NEW MOON

The new moon is quite significant in the Hindu calendar. People generally wait for the new moon to start new works.

The new moon is the beginning of the month in the Chinese calendar.

The new moon signifies the start of every Jewish month and is considered an important date and minor holiday in the Hebrew calendar. ~ Wikipedia

Oh! Sometimes I feel like I am in such perfect and divine alignment with life and Spirit. This is one of those times. I am so present to the beauty and magnificence of life. My heart feels full and expansive, my body open, my breath deep, my mind clear. I feel that feeling of true inner joy that is talked about. A joy of being alive, for being here. A moment of 'delightenment' as my one of my dearest teachers, Donna Martin, calls it. These are precious moments to be cherished and anchored in my being and to be called upon in those times when I face challenge or adversity.

Do you think it's really true that we must experience the lows in order to experience the highs? Is that truly our lot in life? Is there a middle way? Well, of course, I have it on good authority that there is. I think Buddha is a pretty reliable source, wouldn't you say? ;-) But how many actually achieve it? I sometimes wonder if peace actually is the ultimate goal. Wouldn't it be boring? There is a theory, you may have heard of, that we created this existence of life as a game, an opportunity to experience all the many aspects of being and all the facets of life. That we came from nothing and we return to nothing, to peace. If you have never seen Bill Hicks riff on the meaning of life, you absolutely must. (Search "Bill Hicks meaning of life" on YouTube.) He's one of my ultimate heroes. I so admire his ability to boldly express himself without thought of consequence. He truly didn't give a shit what people thought of him.

Being a stand-up comedian is one of my other secret goals in life. That's the ultimate freedom and boldness of expression and the joy of making people laugh! Such a gift. I have had fleeting moments of it when I have led workshops. It's such a wonderful feeling to be able to make someone laugh. Isn't laughter the greatest thing ever? Man, we all need to laugh more. Well, at least I do. I definitely laugh way more than I used to, but there's room for improvement in that area. I think one the greatest accomplishments is to be able to have humour with yourself and with life. I see that as one of the saving graces in relationship, for sure. My dad and stepmother (my second mom), Marilyn, are constantly laughing at themselves and each other, rarely taking each other too seriously and, when they do, they quickly let it go and laugh about it. I see that as being one of the main reasons they've stayed happily married for over twenty-two years. It's a huge inspiration to me. Obviously this is my dad's second marriage, as I'm a little *(okay, quite a lot)* older than twenty, although I don't act it most of the time. ;-)

That's been another of my greatest challenges in life, 'growing up.' Whatever that means. But seriously, for some strange reason, I have resisted truly becoming an adult. I still don't quite support myself. I rely on my parents for support, both financially and emotion- ally. Well, that's not completely true. Last year was the first year in a long time that I didn't live beyond my means! That was a huge accomplishment for me. I guess you could say I'm a late bloomer. ;-) I am making progress. I just haven't understood what this whole life thing is really about. I've had a very difficult time with it to say the least. Being a dreamer, I have had trouble with 'reality.' I don't really understand what reality is yet, either. There are so many different ideas and theories about it. Some say this life is an illusion; some live as if it's very real and take it very seriously. The jury's still out for me on this one. In one of my epiphinal moments during an Enlightenment/ Illumination Intensive, I was working on the koan 'what is life.' I had the realization that "life is to be lived and not contemplated." I laughed so hard when I got that. It was hilarious to me as I'd spent so much of my life in contemplation trying to figure 'life' out. Another epiphany I've had is, "All I can truly know is this moment." Anything else is an idea or a concept. Any ideas of afterlife, reincarnation, returning to the Source are all theory, they come from my mind. Even though I have had flashbacks of previous lives in Clearing sessions. But who's to say that my mind didn't just make that shit up or, at the very least, embellish on it in some way. That's why I come back to "this moment is all I can truly know." This was actually quite liberating and empowering for me because it made me realize that I need to make the most of every moment rather than put off for some unknown, unforeseeable future possibility. I had spent quite some time looking for an escape, an excuse to check out, an opportunity to transcend this miserable existence, as I once thought of it.

CLEARING

Clearing was developed between 1965 and 1975 by an American, Charles Berner. It's based on the observation that inner conflicts and states of unhappiness come about as a result of stuck communications.

Clearing takes place in a one-to-one setting either face-to-face or over Skype. You work in areas of your interest that you would like to untangle and get to go better. The Clearer guides you in communication processes that clear current problems, develop

communication ability, and free inner tensions. Some processes target special problem areas such as depression, maintaining healthy personal boundaries, or improving a group involvement gone bad.

In general, Clearing sessions help you have better relationships and a better sense of yourself. From this, many things go better. You can get on with the life projects you find most important and most true to your heart. Clearing clients often report a sense of release, empowerment, and of coming home to who they really are.[4]

I had a rude awakening, and yet also a liberating moment at another Enlightenment/ Illumination Intensive, when I got that "I am human." This may seem obvious and ridiculous, but you have to understand my state of mind at the time. I was seeking spirituality and enlightenment to escape the human experience. I thought that if I awakened then I could be a spiritual being and be above it all. Isn't that hilarious? The most perfect paradox; one of my awakenings was that I am human, no escaping it. Oddly enough this was quite liberating, as I mentioned, because aspiring to be a spiritual being, I was putting a lot of pressure on myself to be perfect and all-knowing and to achieve miraculous feats. When I realized that I was human, flaws and all, I could give myself space to just be, to make mistakes, and to be human. I didn't have to be perfect anymore and that meant I could let others off the hook and not expect everyone else to be perfect. That was a tortuous way of being for myself and for others. Unfortunately, some of that perfectionism still lingers, but I at least know how to manage it. I have grown my capacity for compassion and acceptance. Of course, there's room for improvement in that area as well, but/and I'm working on it all the time. It may be time to take a break now. I've shared a lot. It feels really good. You have no idea. I've been thinking about writing a book for at least 10 years now. Have had so many ideas for topics and titles, but the inspiration wasn't there. Until now! There's just one more thing I want to share before I go and dance some more.

I had a tarot reading a few weeks back to help get some insight or clarity about my life. I was starting to feel that familiar feeling of discontentment and wondering what I was meant to do with my life. I knew I wasn't going to be a bodyworker and yoga teacher the rest of my life. At least I hope not. I could sense a deeper purpose wanting to emerge, but I had no idea what it was and wanted some assurance or a sign that I was on the right path or, if not, then some sense of which direction to go next. I had only had one other full tarot reading in my life when I was around twenty and didn't really appreciate it back then. I'm often a skeptic and a bit wary of stuff like this, but I kept getting this inkling, this impulse, a voice kept telling me to go. I finally gave into the voice and booked a session with a local tarot reader, Oriane Lee, who I heard on good authority was gifted She was lovely, I instantly felt welcome and at ease in her presence. She had an aura of warmth and kindness. I could sense she actually cared. The reading was brilliant, great affirmations and guiding posts. Perhaps I'll tell you more about it sometime, but I'm too tired right now. The one thing I want to share is that she said by mid-April something would emerge from me that is uniquely my own. Today I wondered if that is this book. That would mean writing it in two months, but it is in the realm of possibility. Time is of the essence. It's been brewing for a long time. Plus I really want to have a child, and all the other possibilities I've explored for creating a nest egg would take too long. That's the Aries in me, I want it now, yesterday. Stubborn and proud of it. So, anyway, we'll see. I'm curious. If not completed then definitely well on its way. Hell, at this rate I may finish by the end of the week! ;-) Tah tah for now.

MY DEEPEST FEAR

I can't sleep. My deepest fear is that I'll die alone and—worse yet—destitute and alone. Having not accomplished anything significant, having no money—a failure. I'm already forty and don't have much to show for it. I'm in debt, and the only thing I really own is a car that's from daddy. I paid for some of it.

About a month before my fortieth birthday, I almost killed myself again, for the third and final time. I was going to say "hopefully final," but then realized it's in my hands—words have power. I didn't even get to the point of attempting it. I was too depressed to even make the effort it would take. I researched it, tried to find the easiest, fastest and most painless way, but it all seemed too complicated, would require too much effort. Instead, I just lay in bed in despair. My life was in shambles, my 'career' had come to an end a few months earlier. All attempts at generating an income failed, no one or very few showed up for my yoga classes; I wasn't getting any sessions, and I had just found out that my partner didn't want to be in relationship with me anymore. My world was falling apart. I was at a loss. I guess I was experiencing a midlife spiritual crisis. Stephen Cope talks about this in his book that I mentioned earlier. I guess it's quite common. Oh yeah, and to top it all off, I was planning a fortieth birthday celebration for myself and getting very little response or interest, was conflicted about whether to cancel it or not, and was facing the loss of at least $800 and my pride. I was feeling very unloved and unsupported, to say the least.

I video logged the whole thing. I had gotten an idea for this project of vlogging every day for the forty days leading up to my birthday. I had this notion that I was going through some profound and powerful transformation and that when I turned forty I would emerge a new and improved being. In some ways, I was right. I didn't realize that I would have to pass through some deep dark territory to get there. The hero's journey, I think they call it. I still have to watch and edit all those. I had intended to create a viewing of some sort, but I'll have to see them for myself first. They may be terrible. But, at the very least, some good material for my book. ;-) I did watch some of it. The first couple days or so, and I remember talking about dealing with some dark force that wanted to take me out. It was all consuming, and I couldn't shake it no matter how hard I tried. I was feeling defeated and hopeless. Deep down there was some knowing that I would make it through. Luckily I did.

I still don't know what that was ... that darkness that overtook me. When I was in it, it seemed so real, and I felt so powerless. I hope and trust that I won't have to face it again. At least if I do, now I know I have the support to get through it. That's how I got through, with the love and support of my family, friends and a few mentors. Luckily my dad was there, and he was very kind and loving. He scooped me up and took me back to Alberta with him. I spent the following weeks in my parents' care. They found a metaphysical healer that I started to see on a regular basis. Because they are even more skeptical than I am, I was shocked and amazed that—of all people—they would send me to him. Marilyn (my second mom) said she had been given his card by her accountant, who had been helped by him through a major health and life crisis. On the day after I arrived, his card kept "jumping out" (those are the words she used) of a book and onto her desk. After the third time, she took it as a sign. They discussed it with me and, at this point, I was willing to try anything.

The healer had supposedly invented some machine that rotated in a certain way and recalibrated your mental and physical condition to one of greater health and well-being. It intrigued me to say the least. I was skeptical but open enough to try. Or should I say 'desperate' enough. I would go to this man's house, lie in his machine for an hour and then have a discussion with him for an additional hour or so. He would ask me questions and mostly he would talk about Lazaris (a channelled being) and his teachings. I would be given the assignment to listen to a Lazaris' talk about a certain topic, such as shame, guilt, love, etc. The talks were fascinating and always included meditations and exercises to do. This went on for about a month. I don't fully understand how they work, but they seemed to help. The essence that I took away from this time spent with this metaphysical healer was the importance of self-love. The most powerful lesson that

I received was that love is an action, and there are seven ways to 'do' love. So I started doing them to the best of my ability.

What to Do for Love and What to Provide for Love[5]

What to Do	What to Provide
Give	Security
Respond	Pleasure
Respect	Vulnerability/Honesty
Know	Trust
Humility to Be	Reduced Fear of Loss
Intimate	Intimacy & Caring
Courage to Commit	Being Known
Care	

LAZARIS

Lazaris says that Love is both a feeling and a state of consciousness, a skill that you can learn and explore. "Love is also an ideal. It is a state of awareness, a state of being or consciousness that you are always seeking. Though you will never fully embrace the totality of Love, in your search, while you stretch and reach, you become more and more of the ideal you pursue. You become more and more the very Love you seek."[6]

At first the process was incredibly difficult. I was so consumed with self-loathing and shame. But eventually, as time went on, the talks worked their magic and as my family's love seeped in, I improved. I also remember being given a book by Abraham Hicks, *Ask and It is Given*, and an important piece in there was the many levels of emotional well-being. Part of my 'treatment' was to start each day determining where I was on the chart, make efforts to get to the next level and to track my progress. I started at the bottom and, by the end of my time in Edmonton, made it to the level of hope and even a hint of enthusiasm. *Another integral part of my treatment was to take time at the end of every day to think of at least five things that I was grateful for. This practice has remained with me and has become an integral part of my life.*

ABRAHAM HICKS EMOTIONAL CHART[7]

1. Joy/Appreciation/Empowered/Freedom/Love

2. Passion

3. Enthusiasm/Eagerness/Happiness

4. Positive Expectation/Belief

5. Optimism

6. Hopefulness

7. Contentment

8. Boredom

9. Pessimism

10. Frustration/Irritation/Impatience

11. Overwhelm

12. Disappointment

13. Doubt

14. Worry

15. Blame

16. Discouragement

17. Anger

18. Revenge

19. Hatred/Rage

20. Jealousy

21. Insecurity/Guilt/Unworthiness

22. Fear/Grief/Depression/Despair/Powerlessness

It was time to return to the coast. I had decided to go ahead with my party and, miraculously, with the help of my dear friend and soul sister, Theda, people were coming. Shaeah's fortieth Birthday Bliss Bonanza weekend story will have to wait. It's time to sleep now. Plus my laptop is about to run out of battery. Time for us both to rest. ;-) Good night.

My fortieth Birthday Bliss Bonanza was a significant event in my life. Some deep and profound healing and transformation happened there that changed the fabric of my being. It was the first time I got on all levels that I was truly loved and supported. About forty of my closest friends and family gathered at a beautiful retreat centre to spend forty hours together sharing, connecting, pampering, celebrating and loving. People were asked to donate money toward the rental. At the end the funds were counted and equalled the exact amount that was needed. If that doesn't help you believe in magic, I don't know what will! ;-)

February 22

A new day has dawned. A brand new day of infinite possibilities as my dear friend and my Lomi Lomi teacher, Wayne Kealohi Powell, would say. What shall unfold today? During my morning meditation, I had a gazillion topics flash through my head of what to share with you. I know a little contrary to the purpose of meditation. It's very difficult for me to achieve a calm clear mind state, but it does happen on occasion.

The two hottest topics on my mind are family and sex, and I don't mean together. Don't get any twisted ideas in your pretty little head. Thank God, I don't have any heart-wrenching stories of abuse or incest. My childhood was challenging enough. Speaking of which, I think I'll start with family. I have a big one, over twenty aunts and uncles. I have countless cousins, so many I don't stay in touch with any of them. In fact, I hardly stay in touch with any of my extended family. I guess I find it too overwhelming. I stay more in touch with my dad's side since there are fewer of them, and they are more connected. My mom's side of the family seemed to be quite close at one time; we would get together often due to weddings, reunions or Christmas and such, but after my grandma died that all fell apart and so did the family. It's quite sad actually. I miss those wild and crazy gatherings.

Speaking of which, I was talking to my crazy aunt Brenda last night, and I mean that in the most affectionate way. She even calls herself that. When I told her I was writing a book, she said—and I quote—"Be sure not to say anything good about your crazy aunt Brenda in there." She's great. I really love her. We have a special bond, I think because I admire her wackiness so much. She's very expressive, her nickname is Motor Mouth and she's proud of it. We had a family tradition, the two of us, at family get-togethers—and there were a lot of them. We would lip-sync Leader of the Pack. My favourite part was the revving of the motorcycle. We would get so into it. It was a hoot. She was a lot of fun *(and still is)*. As a teenager, I would go with her and her family to Shuswap Lake for a week or two in the summer. Those were good times, water skiing, campfires, picnics, stargazing and rye and cokes. Yeah, she was a bit of a bad influence on me. But it was better to get that out of my system with family than on the streets or in bars with strangers.

I got drinking out of my system by the time I was seventeen. I don't even remember going to the bar when I turned eighteen. I'm not saying I didn't partake in alcohol in my adult years; I have a few memorable stories to tell about that, but I'll save those for another time. Anyway, what's my point? I guess there isn't a point. Just sharing. Well, I guess there is a point or maybe just a question. It's about family and the importance of it. I cherish the huge lively festive gatherings we had throughout my childhood, I think it gave me a sense of connection even though a part of me never really felt like I belonged, I was the different one.

Most members of my mom's family were redneck, meat-eating, beer-swilling, hardworking folk, and I was this airy-faery, theatrical, travelling gypsy, vegetarian flower child. It was hilarious actually. I would get teased a lot. Just to give you a clear image of our differences, our family reunions were called 'Pig Roasts,' and I was a vegetarian and part Jewish. Despite our differences, there was a lot of fun had and a lot of love shared. "Salt-of-the-earth" folks, as my dad calls them; they are indeed. I guess my question is, "How important is it to maintain good ties to extended family?"

I'm realizing that I've been avoiding the whole situation with my mom's side of the family. It's quite a mess. At one point I had visions of helping everyone resolve their differences and bring us back to one big happy family, but it's too daunting. And is it my business or responsibility? It could easily take up all of my time and energy. It comes down to how important it is to me. Is it a priority? At this point in my life, no. I have my own life to get together, my own issues to address. Perhaps at some point I'll be ready and willing to put energy there but not now, and I'll have to live with that, even though I know it breaks my mom's heart to have her family so broken. She's the oldest and I sense she feels a certain amount of responsibility. So I listen compassionately and give her as much of my love and energy as I can. My primary family is super important to me. I have put a lot of energy, blood, sweat and tears into repairing, resolving, clearing and improving my relationships with my mom and my dad. My dad especially. That was a huge project and well worth the effort.

I just had a great Surrender Yoga session. I started out similarly to—or actually I mirrored exactly—the way I ended my last session, which was in the fetal position on my left side. I ended my last session in the fetal position on my right side. Very interesting. So I was lying there, and the familiar thoughts started arising: "When's something going to happen?"; "Why isn't anything happening?"; "Oh, God, am I going to just lie here again for the whole hour? I don't want to lie here for an entire hour ..." and so on. At one point, I get this hit: "Gee, maybe there's a lesson here for me." So I start to become curious and sure enough the thought arises, "I need to learn how to just be and not be doing all the time." Then, something amazing happened, I actually let go and surrendered. Go figure.

Just as I was sinking into the surrendering of just being, my lovely monkey mind started asking God/the Divine all these questions, "Well, how am I going to know when to move?"; "Will I ever move?"; "How does it really happen?" And suddenly this voice came through and said, "My will is thy will, you will know, our wills are one in the same." My will = thy will, thy will = my will. It was like a flash of reckoning, but then, of course, I had to question, "Yeah, but what about when I do things wrong or ..." and the voice interrupted me, "My love, you are a child of God, an extension of me. How could anything you do be wrong?" And I crack myself up because at that I said, "Well, see, how could our wills be the same if I'm your child, children also have different wills from their parents, in fact. We make a point of it, we love to rebel ..." Blah blah blah, and then—I'm trying to remember what happened, oh yeah—the wise voice within said, "There is an adult in you that knows ..." or something like that. I can't remember exactly. The gist of it was "Trust yourself, you'll know."

Finally, I let go and rested in the stillness of my being and, at some point, I started to feel an energy generate inside of me, around the area of my heart, and it began to spread; I began to feel excited and intrigued but still didn't move. I lay there feeling and curious about what would happen. And I can't even pinpoint the moment, but the next thing I knew I was moving my body and feeling the sensations, and it felt good. I recalled one of the important components of Surrender Yoga that I learned in my Kripalu training, and I began to repeat the words over and over again, "Breathe relax feel watch allow," and I flowed through various movements and qualities of breath, sometimes pausing and holding a position for a few—or multiple—breaths at times. My movement became like a dance, and all of a sudden the alarm sounded, indicating that my hour was over, and I didn't feel done. I kept going for a while and then, at one point, I felt done so I lay down in shivasana and allowed time for the integration of my experience.

I had forgotten how amazing and powerful Surrender Yoga can be. I could feel my body's own wisdom guiding me, moving me. My body knew what it needed for releasing held tension and pain and for opening and realigning itself. It's quite interesting because I recently started studying Ashtanga Yoga, which is very structured, focussed a lot on proper placement and sequences and is very detailed and specific about how to move in and out of poses. I have been really enjoying that deepened awareness and knowledge of my body and how it works. There is definite benefit in that system, and I will continue to practise it AND I have a renewed interest and commitment to practicing Surrender Yoga as well, in which all knowledge is released and the body becomes the guide. I love how different, and yet complementary, the two practices are. The perfect metaphor for the paradox of life.

KRIPALU YOGA

Kripalu Yoga is a comprehensive, disciplined approach to self-study that cultivates health, facilitates psychological growth, and transforms one's sense of self. Kripalu Yoga arises from thousands of years of study and practice in fostering a spiritual connection to all life and an awakening to the authentic self. It focuses on getting in touch with one's own innate wisdom and happiness through cultivating nonjudgmental awareness. Kripalu means "being compassionate" in Sanskrit, and compassion for oneself and others lies at the heart of Kripalu Yoga.

Kripalu Yoga encompasses three stages of practice, but these stages are not achieved in a linear fashion, like climbing the rungs of a ladder. Rather than a series of steps, the stages represent a cyclical, never-ending process of evolution and learning.

In stage three, often called "meditation in motion," the practitioner is guided primarily by intuitive knowledge and prana (energy, or life force), attuning to the subtle wisdom of the body and spirit. Kripalu Yoga teaches that when we allow ourselves to be guided by this wisdom in every facet of life, our connection with self and with others becomes stronger and deeper, and we experience physical, mental, emotional, and spiritual well-being.[8]

ASHTANGA

Ashtanga is a system of yoga transmitted to the modern world by Sri K. Pattabhi Jois (1915–2009). This method of yoga involves synchronizing the breath with a progressive series of postures—a process producing intense internal heat and a profuse, purifying sweat that detoxifies muscles and organs. The result is improved circulation, a light and strong body, and a calm mind.[9]

Speaking of life, I spent most of my day joyfully cleaning the house, preparing for my mom's return. I had the music blaring and was getting into every nook and cranny, clearing all the dust bunnies and piles of dog and cat hair. I don't think I mentioned that I am at my mom's place in the Peace Country of Northern Alberta, looking after the animals and plants and keeping the fires burning while she's been enjoying a long overdue getaway to Mexico. I love my mom. Tomorrow I pick her up and will be spending another week here with her. She's really an amazing woman. She truly loves me unconditionally; I feel and know that with my whole being, have never doubted it and think that's the most profound gift a parent can give their child or anyone, for that matter. We have always shared a special bond and have gone through our share of challenges and conflicts as well, but the love has been steadfast and true. I know I've hinted at a troubled childhood, but I know how blessed I am to have my mother and her quality of love. Not everyone is as lucky.

I'm feeling a little stuck right now, unsure of which direction to go. To elaborate on my mom or go back and continue where I left off about my dad, or there are thoughts about the family stuff I shared. Instead I'm going to let it rest and let the love of my mom reverberate and permeate through these pages, and I send a blessing out to you that you may be so blessed to feel the quality of love that I have the great honour and privilege to know from my mom.

FEBRUARY 23

I just got home from picking up my mom. We've had a full day of running around the big city of Grande Prairie to get all our supplies for the week. Did I mention that my mom's place is in the boonies? She lives at the end of a dead end road with the nearest neighbour at least a 30-minute walk away. And the nearest town a 20-minute drive. It's a very special place. I'm pretty wiped and not even sure what to say, but I'm keeping to my commitment of writing thirty minutes a day so here goes. Let me pause and take a few minutes to tune in and to reflect on my day. I close my eyes and take a few deep breaths. I can't concentrate because my mom is talking on the phone to my grandpa who just had an operation on his penis, and she's laughing at his stories about his experience. Penis humour. He's just about to turn ninety. He's a real character. More active than most 20-year olds. He still drives, walks a lot, loves to play games and loves to dance. He even still makes things like tinmen out of old cans and wooden signs and animals. My mom's garden is full of them.

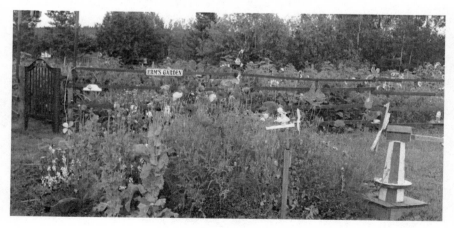

Every time I talk to him, he says he's "keepin' busy," and "gotta keep going." His theory is that, if he stops, he will seize up and won't be able to get up again. Always a big kidder. He lives on white bread, potatoes, meat, coffee and sweets; he's skinny as a stick and has more energy than most people. He and my grandma, when she was alive, were the living version of the nursery rhyme, Jack Sprat …

He threw himself his own ninetieth birthday party, hired his favourite band and danced the night away. He told me he had a really great time. One of my regrets is that I didn't make it to that party. I had an event to work at that weekend and, at that time, my contract was for only seven events a year, and I couldn't afford to miss it. But if I had really wanted to, I could have made it happen, of course. How often does your grandfather turn 90 and throw his own party? Oh well, live and learn. My mom just shared with me that the first night he was home after the surgery, he was having complications and couldn't pee. He was in a lot of pain and had plans to go back to the hospital the next day, but he says in the middle of the night a ghost doctor threw him out of bed and, while he was lying on the floor, he passed a blood clot so he didn't have to go back to the hospital. I said it was probably grandma. They both got a chuckle out of that. Oh, now she's on the phone with Motor Mouth. I can see this may be challenging to write now that she's home. That's okay, tests of commitment are good. Have to be willing and able to work under all conditions, right?

Speaking of commitment, I did a dyad with my friend, Theda, during my hour and a half drive to Grande Prairie. We worked on, "Tell me why you believe you don't have what it takes." The night before, during a coaching conference call for social entrepreneurs who want to grow their business, I had identified this as one of my core beliefs. The dyad was awesome. I love dyads.

DYAD

Dyads are a formal model for communication in which one person is the listener, and one person is the speaker. The listener listens without making any comments or judging in any way. When the speaker is done, the listener says "thank you," and

the roles reverse. It is a powerful and effective way to move through the different layers of the mind to bring ideas, concepts and beliefs to consciousness and to access one's own inner wisdom and truth.

I became clear that the main reasons I hold the belief that "I don't have what it takes" are due to the lack of confidence in myself, my pattern of self-sabotage, my cycle of depression and the fact that I compare myself to others. I think that where I am at is insufficient or 'less than,' and it means that I am a failure. By the last round of the dyad, I actually felt that I don't hold that belief anymore and that—as I mentioned earlier—I am just a late bloomer. Just because others of my age have accumulated a lot more than I have doesn't mean my path is worse or wrong. I am a unique being, and I am finding my way. In fact, deep inside I always knew I would come into my own. Who knows, I could be wrong, and I may die destitute, but I have an inkling that won't be the case. Time will tell.

FEBRUARY 24

Both mom and I have felt tired and lazy today. It's been a cloudy, low-energy day. I did shovel some snow, brought in a load of wood and went for a short walk. There was a bitter wind, so I made it quick. I did my yoga practice, an hour and half of the Ashtanga series. I really had to push myself to start, but once I did, I got into it and at the end I felt great. Now I'm wiped.

Today is the last day of my cleanse, and I'm ready for some real sustenance. Tomorrow I get to move on to juices, woo-hoo! And then the next day, raw fruit and veggies. Mom's been torturing me with her eating. The smells especially get my gastric juices flowing and stomach rumbling. Oh well, it's a great test of my conviction and discipline. All qualities I'm needing to strengthen.

I've been really getting into Stephen Cope's book; it's so perfect for me. He starts out talking about his midlife spiritual crisis and about his journey of coming back to himself during his time at Kripalu. I was reading about transformation, recreating oneself, supportive spaces, direct experience, Samadhi. All things I can relate to, that have been a significant part of my life journey. Something he wrote keeps reverberating in my mind; it was actually a quote from a friend of his, "Any mature adult has more than one church." For some reason this really struck me and resonates with me. I have always struggled with total devotion to one way or one teaching or teacher. At times I have made this mean that there's something wrong with me or that I'm missing out on something. At times, I've even been envious of those who find that one thing that they connect with; I have wondered whether it provides them some extra strength or power that I will never know.

This struggle with devotion also applies to my life purpose. I have always had multiple interests and haven't found any one thing that I specialize in or excel at. As I write this, I realize I'm being hard on myself as my life's work and dedication to spiritual awakening, liberation and to well-being have been quite consistent, and yet I still feel like a novice in that realm. Even with yoga, despite having practised it for over ten years, I feel like I'm just beginning. There's still so much more to learn. Again—as I write this—I realize that this is actually a good thing and perhaps a sign that I have actually learned something. For, in my humble opinion, one of the greatest teachings/learnings on the yogic path is to always be a beginner, to come from beginner's mind.

Something else that's been reverberating through my brain from the conference call I was on a few nights ago was, "We often teach what we most need to learn." It's not the first time I've heard that expression. In fact, I'm very familiar with it and painfully aware of how it's been true in my life. I'm fascinated by how we often think we have to be an expert in something in order to teach it—but, really, I think the most important element is 'authenticity.' Is it something that speaks to your heart, that you have a genuine interest in? And, as I write this, it is coming to me that in fact it may be even better that I don't know everything about something to teach it; otherwise, I end up imposing it on someone rather than evoking their own drive to learn it and, most importantly, to make it their own.

Am I making sense? Sometimes when I share things, I feel like they are coming out in a big jumble and like others may not be able to follow me or to understand what I'm getting at. Oh well, in the editing I'll review it and see if it needs tweaking or not. I have had conflicted ideas about this writing, at times I've considered going back over what I've written and fleshing out certain topics; the other thought is to just leave it as it is so that it doesn't lose the power of its rawness. We'll see, I'll get other's opinions on it, too. I wonder if I will self-publish or get a publisher. I think I will try to get it published by someone else first, just for the fun of it and, if no one wants it, then I'll self-publish.

I had a fun thought the other day that the perfect publisher is a fictional character, Erica Strange, from my favourite TV show, Being Erica. I thought that, if I could find a real live publisher like Erica, she would love it and be all over it. I've set that intention and put it out to the Universe so we'll see what happens. For the first time, I'm actually waiting for the timer to go off and, just as I wrote that, it did. I'm done. Going to do some mindless TV watching with my mom.

FEBRUARY 25

I find myself falling into my pattern again. I'm comparing myself to Stephen Cope and feeling inferior. Thoughts like, "He expresses himself so eloquently and intelligently. Why would anyone want to read what I have to say?"; "His path is more profound"; "He's covering all the topics I want to. Why bother?" Aaaaah! I want to scream with frustration and impatience with myself. This is my expression, this is about me, it doesn't have to be like anyone else's—in fact, it shouldn't. It needs to be unique, it is unique, I am uniquely me and that's okay. In fact, it's great! I am wonderful and beautiful and perfect just as I am. I feel sadness now, for doubting myself, for that slight betrayal to my own being. Why do I do that? Where does that come from? And why? I don't know, and it doesn't matter. What matters is that I pick up and start again despite the voices of doubt, fear and criticism. That's what one of my teachers said a true master is, "Not someone who is perfect or does everything perfectly, but one who doesn't let anything take them out, that each time you fall down you get up and start again. That's the sign of a true master." I heed those words to the best of my ability. Over and over and over and over again. Believe me, I have fallen what seems like countless times. So far, no matter how hard or far I've fallen, I've gotten up and started again. Sometimes a little—or very—bruised and sore. I may take some time to hide out and lick my wounds, but eventually I re-emerge hopeful, willing, open and optimistic, and I like to think, a little wiser. ;-)

I think one of the most challenging aspects—or I guess more aptly, 'choices'—after a fall or a setback is to stay open. One can easily let life's hard knocks shut you down. I have met some very closed and jaded people, and I can understand why; life can hurt, but I still find it sad and unfortunate. Personally, one of my greatest commitments and life missions is to keep opening my heart, to choose love instead of fear. And, in that department, I can honestly and proudly say I have succeeded, am succeeding. It's an ongoing practice and commitment. So I may not have a house, RRSPs or have accumulated worldly goods, but I have an open, loving and compassionate heart and, to me, that is worth more than any money or material gain I could ever acquire.

I have made my relationships my priority. I was reflecting last night about how this visit with my family is a testament to my practice and to the work that I've done. It's been the best visit ever. Some say that if you meet a person who claims to be awakened, a surefire test of the degree to which they are living their enlightenment is to ask them about their relationship to their mother. My test is the relationship with my father. I do not by all means claim to be enlightened but, if medals were given for the transformation of one's relationship to their parents, I would win the platinum gold. I let out a little chuckle at this one. Yeah, I do like to blow my own horn sometimes. Why not, I've worked hard and, in my mind, it's a huge accomplishment. Like every great award winner, I have to admit that I couldn't have done it alone. I had a lot of help from family, friends and professionals.

As much as I find Stephen Cope's writing intimidating and challenging so do I find it as equally, if not more so, affirming and inspiring.

I sit in my mom's recliner next to the burning fire and the glow of the TV. I've been sitting here for hours; I have a headache and my eyes are tired and sore, and yet I can't pull myself away. This is why I have never owned a TV. I spent a lot of my childhood watching TV. It was my favourite form of escapism, second after books and the other, long walks in the woods with my faithful companions, Belle and Digger. I feel like I've regressed to that little girl. It often or, more honestly, always happens when I visit my parents. To some degree or another. I think it's probably natural and happens to a lot if not most people. Misery loves company. ;-)

February 26

I was watching the Oscars, and they had just gotten to the best leading actor when our power went out! Talk about terrible timing. I'm a sucker for Hollywood. I love the glamour, the fashion, the sparkle, the entertainment.

I haven't mentioned that one of my biggest dreams was to be a movie star. In fact, at one point in my life, I was convinced I would be one. I went to a performing arts high school—during which time I won an award for some competition for a monologue that I did, got a paid part in a TV commercial, was a poster girl for our school and got the leading role of Titania in our year-end show. I took singing lessons, dance lessons, voice lessons, and speech lessons. I was a small town girl looking to make it big.

I started my BA in Drama at the University of Alberta with the intention of getting into the BFA Acting Program, one of Canada's best acting programs. I had ambition, drive and hutzpah, but I guess not enough, 'cause I never got into the program. I auditioned two years in a row and, for some reason, I gave up after that. And at some point during my degree, I gave up on acting all together and resorted to being a stage manager—even though during those first couple years of university I acted in quite a few shows. Was even one of the few BAs to be in one of the BFA's showcase plays. But at some point, my spirit broke and I gave up.

In a Clearing session that I had a couple years ago, I realized that the point when I gave up on my dream of being an actor and being a movie star was the day I gave up on myself. That was a hard blow to take. For many years, I had blamed it on my parents, for not believing in me, for not being more supportive. In my memory, my dad and my second mom were always trying to convince me to be more practical, to become a nurse or a teacher. Recently I talked to them about this, and they said that they were very supportive. Who knows what's real? I don't know what really went down, it was a crazy time.

Around that time, I had moved out of my parents' house and moved in with a man I had 'fallen in love with.' Let's call him George. We were together a few months when I discovered he was some sort of sociopath and had lied to me about almost everything (heritage, profession, finances, etc.). I found out when an eviction notice was slid under our door and the phone bill came with over $300 in phone-sex charges. I asked my biker friend to come over that same day while George was at work and we moved everything out. Luckily I found a pile of cash under the bed to cover the phone bill.

I moved back into my parents' place; I had nowhere else to go. I was utterly ashamed, especially because my dad had told me it was a bad idea to move in with George. I hated proving him right and leaving him to gloat with that "I told you so."

I became really depressed, and my doctor put me on Prozac for a while until I fainted in the shower. I went off Prozac but continued with the counselling. A good friend of mine had died a tragic death during that time as well. It's hard to keep it all straight—what happened when and why or how. One thing was clear, I needed to escape.

The next year I applied for an exchange program that took me to Winchester, England for 8 months. It was a documentary filmmaking course. I loved it. It was foreign, different, exotic, exciting, challenging. True to form, I joined the rugby team and ended up dating a rugby player, who nicknamed himself Puck and me Titania. To this day he writes me little notes of well wishes from Puck to Titania. My life has often paralleled that of a faery tale.

The faithful dreamer that I am; a line from the Oscars tonight made me feel that I still may have a place in Hollywood. Something about 'it takes a big dreamer to be a great director.' I have tons of ideas for movies and TV shows. Well, maybe not tons, but a few. I'm curious to see if any of my visions will actually manifest into reality. I meant my visions for film and TV, but I am curious about all of my visions. I have managed to manifest some of my visions but not many. Manifestation is another of my ongoing challenges. Which seems strange for a woman with so much fire but, for some reason, I can get easily discouraged or distracted. I can be as equally stubborn though and can defy all odds. I guess it depends on the circumstances.

I kind of feel like I'm jumping all over the place and fear that I am not going deep enough. Just skimming the surface so to speak. I'm not sure if that's because I'm avoiding anything or just because that's just where the flow of my thoughts are taking me. I'm sure I'll get deeper as I go. For now I'm just giving you little tastes, little morsels of my life's journey and, as we progress, we'll sink deeper into the meat and bones. We are just getting to know each other after all. ;-) Don't want to give too much of myself away too quickly. Have to keep you intrigued and wanting more, right?

FEBRUARY 27

Supposedly I am over-identified with my body, according to yogic philosophy. I've known this for a long time. I came close to de-identifying from my body once, during an Enlightenment/ Illumination Intensive. I could feel the roots of synapses pulling away from the connective tissue. It was exquisitely painful and liberating at the same time, but I think my mind got in the way and I stayed connected. I couldn't let go, even though I desperately wanted to, maybe that's why. My experience is that I can't escape or get past something until I fully experience it, especially if I don't want to. 'The way out is through,' so they say. I think that's a big part of my karma, to fully embrace and experience the physical before I can be free of it.

According to Gregor Maehle's book, *Ashtanga Yoga*, part of the attachment to the physical also manifests in the ways we relate to the material world and to our families. Material gain hasn't been that important to me, but family definitely is. Materialism is a sign or symptom of our times. We're in Phase 4 of yogic history called The Age of Technology where most people suffer from an 'infatuated mind' (mudha chitta). Maehle wrote, "Infatuated here means obsessed with one's own body, wealth, appearance, and family relations."[10] I guess I actually fit the bill in all four obsessions. Even though I haven't accumulated wealth or put a lot of energy towards it, my mind definitely obsesses over it at times, fantasizes of the possibility of being wealthy, 'financially free,' someday. Have you read the book, *Siddhartha* by Herman Hesse? If not, it's something else I strongly recommend as it fits well with this theme.

FEBRUARY 28

Today was a good day. This morning I asked my mom what could we do together that is fun. We pulled out the clay and had a pottery day. It was awesome. I ended making a really funky phallic flower chalice with a heart-shaped base. I am quite pleased with it. The second piece I made was a flower-petal dish. I love working with clay; there's something very satisfying about squishing earth between my fingers and being able to create form out of nothing. I think all my years of massaging bodies has made my hands sensitive to molding form.

A few years ago when I was here at my mom's, I pulled out a big hunk of clay and, by the end of the evening, I had created a man and a woman intertwined in a passionate embrace. It was my first attempt at sculpting ever. I felt like I was born to sculpt. I bought clay and supplies when I went home with intentions to keep sculpting. I've only made one other sculpture since. Until now. It's an ongoing theme in my life: to get really excited about something and to think it's going to be my life's calling and then very quickly the excitement fizzles out. A part of me thinks, "Hey, that's natural, ebb and flow, no biggie." Another part of me thinks it's a symptom of my deficiency.

I'm not liking my writing these days. I hear my inner critic telling me what shit this is and how no one is going to want to read this. I stay firm to my commitment and keep writing anyway. That's what editing is for. ;-)

Earlier today on my walk, I was wondering what would have happened if I'd never given up on my dream of being an actor. How would life be different? At times I'm convinced that if I'd maintained the level of certainty I had of becoming a movie star, I would have. But who can truly say? The reality is that I allowed external influences to dissuade me from my goal, and I made the choice to quit. I trust and know it's what needed to happen because it did. I needed to go on the path that I chose. I needed to explore the depths of my soul and deepen my experience of life. My soul was calling me to another destiny that has yet to unfold, is in the process of unfolding. My life has been rich with incredible experiences. I wouldn't change it, although at times I would have claimed otherwise. I have definitely had my moments of weakness, where I have begged God for mercy. But at this time, I am content, grateful and happy.

It's amazing how challenging it is to be content, at least for me. Another one of my greatest challenges. I have had an incessant need to seek deeper, fuller, greater, more. I have had a restless soul most of my life. Hence, the wandering gypsy that I've been. I noticed myself getting restless yesterday. It's so difficult to just be still and not do much. And yet I also seem to have a tendency to be lazy. I will avoid doing things that I know I need or want to do and instead distract myself with Internet, emails, movies, food or daydreaming.

I am feeling juvenile in this moment—the inner critic telling me that my writing is a mess, all over the place, not saying much, jumping around the bush, nonsense—but I don't care. It doesn't matter. It's not the point to be brilliant every moment of every day. The point is to keep writing, keep my commitment, keep the juices flowing and, amidst the drivel and drab, will be the odd gem or hopefully many gems. Who knows. It was amazing actually, that during my clay play time, the inner critic didn't come out, and I was actually able to just play and create without that voice telling me it was bad or wrong or silly. It's a wild and very imperfect piece I created and I love it. Often when I begin to create, that voice will come in and try to interfere with the creative process.

MARCH 1

**Love begins at home, and it is not how much we do ...
but how much love we put in that action.
~ Mother Teresa**

I'm on the plane to Vancouver from Edmonton; the sun is setting and a beautiful bright orange glow emanates across the horizon. My heart is a mix of sadness and excitement. Sad to leave my mom, probably to not see her again for at least six months. Excited to be going home, to discover what awaits. Potential romance, new opportunities, musical and artistic exploration. I'm homesick. I yearn desperately to wake up in my own bed, have my own space, the freedom and time to do my practices of yoga, dance, meditation, writing, walks in nature. I'll miss my daily walk with the dogs and, of course, the cuddles with Tuk Tuk *(one of the dogs)* and China *(one of the cats)*. Mom's pets are such bundles of love. A testament to her nature.

I feel sadness, and I'm not sure exactly what about. Tears well up. My heart feels heavy. During our final embrace before we parted ways, my mom whispered in my ear, "We live too far apart." She also said, "I'm an Alberta girl and you're a BC girl." That's just the way it is.

But the sadness feels deeper than that, like I'm not only leaving behind my mom but also a piece of myself. I guess I had expectations for my time there; I had hoped I would 'find myself' more deeply and fully. I was hoping for an experience of 'truly coming home to myself.' I had a flash of it, but I feel that I didn't go deep enough. Somehow I just skimmed the surface and didn't connect to my core as deeply as I had hoped. When mom came home, I felt like I progressively lost touch with myself, merged more with her—like a chameleon—changed my shape and my way of being to match hers. This was partly intentional, to create affinity and to connect, but some of it was involuntary, unconscious and habit.

Yesterday I realized at midnight that I hadn't done my writing, I had a choice to do it or to let it go. I chose to let it go, reasoning that I chose to dedicate that last day to my mom, and I feel okay about that. More sadness arising. Not sure why. More tears. Spilling over now, falling down my face. I sigh with the feeling of release. What is it? Grief? Loss? Letting go? Lost opportunity?

It was a good visit, sweet, comfortable. I was helpful; we accomplished all that we set out to do. Mom always has a list of things to do, and we did everything on that list and then some, but what did I contribute from myself? I didn't originate much contribution. We did do facials, but I usually offer to brush her hair or massage her shoulders or feet. I didn't this time. Why not? Why was I holding back? I did ask her to join me for yoga a couple times and once she did join in. It just never feels like enough: I didn't offer enough, we didn't talk about enough things, we didn't do enough. More sadness, hurt, disappointment in myself. More tears. My heart aches. Maybe it's the loneliness I felt for her, being there all alone. But she has her amazing pets and great friends. I don't know. Maybe it's just that we are different, and I'm coming to terms with that. Or maybe that we are similar, and I'm coming to terms with that. Or both.

We're flying over the Rockies now, so stunning, majestic, timeless. More sadness. Thoughts of wishing that we had shared more affection, that we had cuddled as much as Tuk Tuk and I did. Why is it that we can share more affection with animals than with each other? I had wanted to ask her why we didn't share much affection. We don't avoid it. Every night we'd share a big hug and kiss goodnight and tell each other we love each other. But I was wondering why we don't cuddle. She shared with me that she had a major breakdown at age forty. That was the year I left home. She said it was horrible. Probably the worst year of her life. I felt bad, but she knows I had to go. Is it enough just to be with someone? To just offer companionship, to be there to listen and share or to simply be?

The tears are flooding now, I can't make them stop. It's good in a way. If I was on my own, I suspect I'd be sobbing. But alas, it's a full flight, and I don't feel comfortable letting go here. She is an amazing woman, so strong, so generous. It amazes me that she can live there on her own. Such a huge responsibility. Maybe these are good tears.

Not that there are bad ones, but I mean that they are a cleansing, an opening, a softening. Rather than thinking that there's a deficiency. The tears just are. It's okay and good to cry. Even if it's on a plane with one hundred or so other people. There's no shame in crying. They really won't stop, they just keep flowing. Deep breaths and enjoy it. Enjoy the humanity of it. It's quite fascinating really, I have no idea why I'm crying so much.

I was just reading a chapter about when relationships end in another book I've been reading, *How to Be an Adult in Relationships,* by David Richio. He talked about the importance of grieving, letting go and acknowledging our humanity, our need for connection and the desire to have our needs met. He talks about five needs in particular that all start with A: Acceptance, Allowing, Affection, Attention and Appreciation. According to him, we feel loved when these five needs are met.

I definitely don't want to repeat my patterns from past relationships. I like to think I'm ready to create a conscious loving relationship that lasts. One based on honesty, trust, respect, love, commitment, awareness, affection, appreciation, humour, understanding, passion, creativity, acceptance and support. It is said that our beliefs create our reality or at least our experience of reality. I know this to be at least partially true. I know that my limiting beliefs can restrict or block certain experiences, and yet surprising and miraculous things happen all the time. I don't think there are any hard-and-fast rules in life. I think the one guarantee in life is that there will always be surprises. I'm constantly trying to navigate the balance between will and surrender, wondering how much of my life is within my control and figuring out what I am supposed to let go of and to give up to the Higher Power.

The sky is crimson now as we sail above white fluffy clouds.

MARCH 5

CORTES ISLAND, BRITISH COLUMBIA

I'm finally home, home sweet home. It feels really good to be here. It feels right. I'm home. It's been quite a whirlwind of events. A few very full days in Vancouver. So much has happened that I don't know where to start. One thing is that I haven't kept my commitment to writing. I became too caught up in the city whirl. I was only going to stay one night, but I got sucked in and ended up staying three nights. It's amazing how badly I wanted to get home. I don't remember feeling that homesick for a long time. I did do some fun things in the city though and, of course, spent way too much money.

While waiting for my connecting flight in the Edmonton airport, I had arranged with my friends to meet up in Vancouver. They had suggested we have dinner together. My thoughts instantly went to my favourite restaurant, East is East, but I didn't say anything and thought we'd discuss it once I arrived. Moments later I get a text from my friend suggesting East is East. I love syncronistic moments like that. Then when I was coming out of the SkyTrain station in Vancouver my friends pulled up at the exact moment I walked out of the station. Giving me that sense that I was in the zone and the flow of life. Off we went to East is East. We had a long wait, but it was so worth it. I absolutely love that place, and they had a live gypsy jazz band, so we were entertained. They also gave us free dessert for waiting so long. We had quite the feast. The whole event was quite magical actually.

The next day I met an old boyfriend I hadn't been in touch with for over five years. It was my most tumultuous relationship, and it hadn't ended well. Due to some odd circumstances, he contacted me a few days before I was due to return to Vancouver and invited me to lunch the next time I was in town. Intrigue, curiousity and the desire to achieve some reconciliation, I responded and agreed to meet. I'm glad I did. We had a delightful time sharing and getting reacquainted. It was healing to be together in a way that was respectful and honouring. He even bought me a gift of a mouth harp.

The afternoon and early evening was spent with my godson, Gabriel, and my friends, his parents. I consider them my extended family, and every time I go to Vancouver, my first priority is to spend time with them. I am totally in love with Gabriel. It was love at first sight, and I pronounced myself to be his godmother. We have a very special bond that I cherish, and I try to spend as much time as I can with him, which his parents greatly appreciate as it gives them a break from the exhausting challenges of parenthood.

I'm starting to think that this is becoming too much like a journal, and I'm losing the juice that I had when I started this writing. But I've been away for a while and have had lots of distraction, so I have to give myself some grace and time to get back into the swing of things. I don't want to just share about the things I did, an account of my activities; I want to speak about what's happening in my heart. It's almost like it's an avoidance of sharing from my heart, safer, less vulnerable.

During my time in Vancouver, my heart was a bit heavy, troubled, unsettled, restless, yearning, dissatisfied. I kept busy enough, but I had difficulty staying present and fully enjoying myself as much as I know I could have. But having said that, I had some rich and quality times. I spent time with people that are important to me. I even had a passionate encounter with a beautiful man, who seduced me and ravished me through the night and into the morning. I went to a play that my friend, Leslie, was in called *Doubt,* which had won a Pulitzer Prize. It was a profound play, very deep and heart wrenching. I was quite affected and deeply moved. I went out for tea with Leslie, someone I had met at the SARK workshop last summer. She's a very inspiring woman. She introduced me to the Transformation Game, which is very powerful. She's a powerhouse, gorgeous, dynamic, talented, charismatic. She's training to be a bikini competitor. She's almost inspired me to do it. I'm seriously considering it as it's so outside my box, would push me beyond my comfort zone and give me the level of challenge I think my body and psyche are craving. We'll see. It's a very far stretch, but it could be quite fun.

My soul sister, Theda, and I took the ferry to the island together so that I could visit her father, stepmom and sister. I had never met her father, even after ten years of friendship with her. She's like a second daughter to my parents. They adore her. I enjoyed finally meeting her family, and we had a lovely visit. Her dad is really into Sabian symbols, so he did my chart. My symbol is supposedly a man and a woman with a winding snake. The interpretation is quite complicated so I'm not sure what it means exactly. I'll recount some of the things that stand out from the overall reading. My chart was very balanced, a good spread of energy throughout the planets. Travel was predominant, partnership important. I actually can't remember anything else. I was so exhausted I obviously didn't absorb much of the information. It was fun though, the family sitting around the fire while he read from his Sabian symbol book about all of our different symbols. Quite sweet.

That night, we watched Woody Allen's newest film, *Midnight in Paris*. Brilliant film, very clever and insightful. Then we watched a heart-wrenching film, *50 First Dates*, which surprised me. It starred Adam Sandler. I didn't expect such a deep and moving film, and I bawled at the end. Today I made my way home, stopped for groceries in Campbell River and made the 4:30pm ferry to Quadra, which meant I'd make it home before dark. While in the ferry line-up, someone I know from the Lakehouse Learning Centre asked me for a ride. I was happy to be of service. We spent the entire trip talking about youth, education or, more accurately, un-schooling. It was fascinating, affirming and inspiring. She's very passionate and can speak clearly and convincingly about the virtues of free school. I was captivated the entire two hours that we were together and could have listened for many more hours. She affirmed all of my suspicions, that allowing children to develop on their own with support, love and encouragement results in them emerging as their brilliant self-empowered selves.

MARCH 6

Whew, what a day. So great to be back. Nothing beats that feeling of being home. That feeling of belonging, ease and flow. Being able to just be myself, comfortable in my own skin, no pretense. That feeling of connection, family, community. One of the best feelings in the world. I spent the morning taking care of business and getting settled back in to my home. I was going to go to Lakehouse, to volunteer, but I realized that I needed to get grounded first. It worked out perfectly because in the afternoon I ended up spontaneously meeting up with the Lakehouse gang down at the beach where I joined them for a rousing game of 'Catch the Flag.' A wonderful way to spend a sunny afternoon. It was really great for everyone to be active and have fun as the community has been shaken by a tragic accident in which a teenage boy was killed in a car crash just a few days ago. The teachers happen to be on strike this week so the students don't have a place to gather and grieve. Talk about poor timing. I didn't know the boy or his family, but I can feel the strain on everyone on the island. When a community is so small, it's practically impossible not to be affected by anything major that happens. A sure sign how connected we truly are.

It was so great to be with the kids and connect in that playful way. The perfect follow up to my conversation with my friend yesterday. I had told her how awkward I had felt when I'd gone to the Learning Centre, not sure of what to do. She told me that the best thing is to just be with the kids and play with them. She said that kids will totally put up a wall if anyone tries to impose anything on them. "Be with them, get interested, ask them what they want to do." She told me amazing stories of her experience with free schooling and the ways that children she has known blossomed into their own brilliance without the restrictions of formal education. It's appalling how our society has become so stifling to the human spirit. I don't understand how or why systems that don't support the well-being of people and the planet seem to prevail. Especially when the alternatives seem so simple and obvious. I guess it's just a sign of our times, there's a greater emphasis on material gain than on the well-being of people and the planet. Hopefully we are evolving or shifting out of it.

I wonder if consciousness will shift during my lifetime. Will there be a mass awakening? At times it seems so possible and—at other times—hopeless. Especially when I watch TV and see what the majority of people are being influenced by and how they spend their time. At the same time, I am seeing more shows about supernatural abilities, alternative realities and human issues. It's fascinating to wonder. Anything is truly possible. I always have to have hope, otherwise I would see no point in living, although ... life is getting more enjoyable.

I still haven't figured out what the meaning of life is. Every time I think I possibly have, something comes along to blow it out of the water. Some of the theories have been: to be happy, to contribute to others, to be of service, to love, to realize our potential, to keep growing, learning and expanding into the possibilities of being, to find inner peace, to accept others and the world as it is. I don't know. It's all so confusing. Maybe it's all of the above. I'm exhausted and need to sleep now.

March 7

I'm feeling particularly exhausted today. I think I've over exerted myself. My body aches all over, and my head is even achy and feels foggy. I still had a pretty good day though, somewhat productive. I did some work on promotion for my offerings, put up posters, created a Facebook group for my Cortes Offerings and created events for my yoga classes, meditation and radio show. I had my first yoga class of the season today. Three people showed up, and they greatly appreciated and enjoyed the class. I was hoping more people would come, but it's a challenging time for everyone. Hopefully more will come next time.

I did my budget today, and I'm not in a great situation. I'm going to probably have to take a cash advance from my credit card to make it through to May when I start working again at Hollyhock. I really need to come up with another source of income. I'm tired of living hand to mouth. I'm looking at making a yoga video. I just need to find the people to help me do it. I have no idea what to budget for it. I just put a posting on the Kripalu Teacher's Group Page to ask if anyone had any advice about it. I've asked a woman I know that has been coordinating youth filmmaking on the Island, and she said she could hook me up with some contacts. So I just have to keep putting energy and to take action towards it, and it'll happen. It's another thing I've been talking about for years.

This year feels like a year of action for me; perhaps it being the year of the dragon has something to do with it or simply that I'm forty and have nothing to show for it, and I'm sick of it. I can no longer ignore that burning desire to be a source of greater contribution to the world. I've mentioned before that I have resisted growing up and don't even really know what 'growing up' means. Well, that's not exactly true. What I've come to realize is that growing up simply means taking full responsibility for my life. Being at cause and authoring my own existence. For some reason, I spent most of my life as a victim, holding others responsible or even ransom for my happiness. Of course, that didn't work and, in fact, only resulted in more misery. The more I take responsibility for my life, the happier I become and, oddly enough, the freer I feel. I have a cousin that calls me a 'free spirit,' which I like to think she is right about. But I have to admit that a part of my flying about and travelling around the world was perhaps an avoidance tactic. I do still want to travel but not as much as I want that feeling of home.

I realized last night after I finished writing and went to bed that I have been critical of my writing as of late because I think I should be espousing profound insights and entertaining stories rather than just reporting about the mundane events of my life. But alas, the mundane is a part of life, a big part of life and should not be under estimated. It's not what we do but how we do things, right?! I am definitely feeling very grateful and blessed to have the life I have. I have become happier now that my life is simpler than ever before. I love walking out my door into nature and taking a short jaunt to the local coop where everybody knows my name. I love being greeted with a smile and a hug and being told that they are happy to see me or glad that I'm back. It's a great feeling. That's the feeling of community. Unfortunately, I think it's an experience that most people lack.

I watched a video on Youtube today about the Occupy Movement by Velcrow Ripper and Ian Mackenzie, who are making a movie called *Occupy Love*. The featured speaker, Charles Eisenstein, who wrote *Sacred Economics*, talks about the direction the world needs to go in, which is about more connectivity, care, respect and, of course, ultimately love. He speaks of a world that works for everybody, a world of healing, a world of peace. He speaks of the cost of material gain and power, which is the loss of connection, the loss of intimacy and the loss of meaning. He says that our economy is set up in a way that we don't need anybody, and this does not promote community: "Joint consumption doesn't create intimacy, only joint creativity and gifts create intimacy." He then goes on to talk about how each individual has an important and necessary gift to give. It's interesting how this ties in to my question about the meaning of life that I asked yesterday; it's almost as if the Universe guided me to this video. He talks about the shift of consciousness being more towards our heart's calling, which is to be of service, to give. He says, "Love is the felt experience of connection to another being." I absolutely love the following line:

> The economist says that more for you is less for me, but the lover knows that more for you is more for me, too. If you love someone, their happiness is your happiness, their pain is your pain, your sense of self expands to include other beings. That's love, love is the expansion of the self to include the other. That's a different kind of revolution, there's no one to fight, there's no evil to fight, there's no other in this revolution. Everybody has a unique calling, and it's really time to listen to that, that's what the future is going to be, it's time to get ready for it and to help contribute to it and make it happen.[11]

Okay, I couldn't stop. Everything that he says at the closing of the video is brilliant and totally in alignment with my vision and my heart's longing. It's exciting to hear and connect with more and more individuals who share the same vision and calling. The Internet is a brilliant tool for that. It's fascinating to wonder what direction the world will take.

I also watched a video about a young girl who gave a talk at the United Nations quite a few years ago, expressing her fears, concerns and desires about our future. It was very inspiring. It's amazing that the direction seems so clear to so many of us, even a 13-year old, and yet the powers that be are doing nothing about it or even seem to be moving in the opposite direction. I don't understand how this world got so screwed up. Is it all truly just a game? Does none of it truly matter? I guess what's important is that it matters to me. It matters that there be justice for all and clean air and water for our future generations. It matters that all life be respected and honoured. It matters to me that we take care of and be kind to each other. It matters that I do whatever I can to contribute to others and to the world in a positive way, that I contribute to the well-being of others and the planet. My life purpose is to love and give as fully as I can for as long as I can. And it's nice to know that others share that purpose. As long as that's the case, there's definitely hope and a life worth living.

MARCH 8

We've all been given a gift, the gift of life.
What we do with our lives is our gift back.
~ Edo

Another amazing day in paradise. So full and diverse. I started the day with Yoga Nidra, nauli, a dance and a smoothie.

YOGA NIDRA

The literal translation of Yoga Nidra is Yogic Sleep. It is an ancient form of meditation that will take you into the deepest levels of relaxation while still remaining fully aware. In this deep state beyond ordinary waking consciousness, you naturally re-align with spirit, allowing you to effortlessly disengage from restrictive physical, mental and emotional patterning. Here, you are free to create a life that is an expression of higher consciousness rather than acquired conditioning.[12]

Yoga Nidra has been a huge blessing in my life. After learning it from Amrit Desai when he came to Hollyhock, I stopped having menstrual cramps, so I bought a few of his CDs and often start my day with it.

NAULI

A yogic cleansing exercise, or kriya. Nauli cleanses the internal organs and tones the abdominal region via a side-to-side rolling motion of the abdominal muscles.[13]

This is a really great practice for anyone with digestive issues.

Then I went to Qi Gong at the hall. I love Qi Gong; it's so comprehensive and holistic. I knew implicitly that I was doing good for my body, my mind, my heart and my spirit. I remember thinking about how some people think it's important to be committed to only one form of practice, and I can't help but think they are missing out, but who's to say what I'm missing out on by not committing solely to one practice. I just love diversity. We are such complex and diverse beings it only makes sense to explore numerous modalities. To me anyway. I already do a bit, but I'd like to bring more Qi Gong into my yoga practice and classes. They complement each other well.

QI GONG

Qi Gong (literally "Life Energy Cultivation") is a practice of aligning breath, movement and awareness for exercise, healing and meditation. With roots in Chinese medicine, martial arts and philosophy, Qi Gong is traditionally viewed as a practice to cultivate and balance qi (chi) or what has been translated as "intrinsic life energy." ~ Wikipedia

I love fusion. I think that's what allows for the uniqueness and authenticity of our own expression rather than just a carbon copy of what someone else has done. Something comes uniquely from us when we allow the merging and blending of all that we have learned and experienced and when we offer that as our gift. I am still exploring and discovering what that is for me. My unique blend of offering. I would have to muster a lot of courage to do that. I have always admired and even envied those that have created their own unique offering and go for it. I'm not sure if I have a lack of confidence or a lack of clarity that has prevented that for me. I think it's a combination of the two, but I honestly haven't had the great inspiration of something to offer that is uniquely mine yet. I have always felt that it is coming. I'm still in the gestation period or, as I have mentioned before, perhaps it's this book. But I feel there's something else, something that's more dynamic and engaging. I am such a physical and sensual being after all. There must be an active form of my offering too, or perhaps it's a package of various things. Like a body of work: my writing, my painting, my music, my dance … that's why I like the idea of my one-woman show because it provides the stage for all of these pieces to be expressed together. It feels too disjointed having all the pieces separate from each other. Maybe it doesn't matter what the presentation is. It's just a preference; each form of offering is a part of me after all. Maybe it's me that is still feeling a bit disjointed. That rings true! ;-)

Oh yeah, so getting back to my day. After Qi Gong was breakfast and then I spent the better part of the day catching up on my book-keeping and even did my taxes. I felt great getting that done. It was about three o'clock when I finished and by then I had been in front of the computer for about three hours. My brain was mush and the sun was peeking out so I decided to go for a walk. I took my favourite route, by the lake over to the waterfall and along the lagoon to the ocean and through the woods back to town. Doesn't that sound great? Again it fulfills my need for diversity. I enjoy standing at the edge of the lake soaking in the calm and peace of its stillness, drinking in the colours of the trees and the sky reflected in the glassy surface of the water. Then I make my way to the vibrant rush of the waterfall, sit there soaking up the negative ions and ozone in the air as I feel the vibration of the pounding water on the earth.

NEGATIVE IONS

Negative ions are odorless, tasteless, and invisible molecules that we inhale in abundance in certain environments. Think mountains, waterfalls, and beaches. Once they reach our bloodstream, negative ions are believed to produce biochemical reactions that increase levels of the mood chemical serotonin, helping to alleviate depression, relieve stress, and boost our daytime energy.[14]

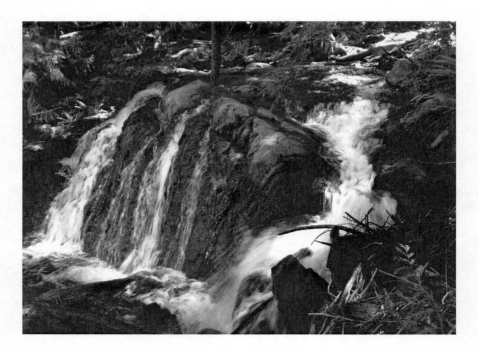

My thoughts flood out and away like the flowing water, clearing my mind. Then I make my way around the edge of the lagoon, transitioning from fresh water to salty ocean. Birds abound. I walk around the point of the spit to finally gaze upon the expansive horizon beyond the anchored boats and the snow-capped mountains framing the distance. I sit on a driftwood log on the beach drinking

From My
Heart
To Yours

in the warmth and energy of the sun before I enter the woods and become engulfed by the mass of the towering trees and thick underbrush. The trail makes its way up a steep incline, just enough to raise my pulse and break a sweat. A few larger cedars and Douglas firs stand like guardians amongst second-growth forest. The sun streams through the branches in rainbow sprays of light. At a couple of vantage points, the trees make way for a breathtaking view of the ocean and horizon below.

This walk makes me happy and is good for me on all levels. It clears my head, oxygenates and strengthens my body. I relax and feel an increased sense of connection and openness. When I walk, I start to feel like everything is okay or at least going to be okay. I remember thinking at some point during the walk that it's a huge source of inspiration because I was getting excited about my book and about writing again. I must remember to get out and walk before I sit down to write. It's almost like it provides the space and time to integrate my experiences and also to connect to the greater consciousness—'tap in,' so to speak.

Oh yeah, and then after my walk, I went to meet a friend and started to build my 'secret garden.' It's so exciting. I haven't had a real garden for at least twelve years. Last year I planted a few plants in my boyfriend's backyard, but I wasn't really around to tend it. We still got tons of peas and zucchinis though. It's incredible how simple it is to grow your own food. One of my greatest thrills is to eat locally grown food; to eat food I've grown myself is beyond … I'm at a loss for words. Simply beyond! I can't wait. I feel like I'm bursting out of my skin with excitement and anticipation. I have a perma-grin on my face as I write this. I sigh with the joy of living my life in alignment with my values. It's been a long time coming. I can honestly say that I am finally living my life in full integrity. Walking my talk, exploring my passions and interests, living my joy, doing what I love. I am definitely the happiest I have ever been, most content and excited about life and its possibilities. The last piece of the puzzle for me is a partner, someone to share my life and my love with. I have so much love to give. There is someone I am seeing. He's a definite potential, but it's still very fresh and new. We are just getting to know each other. We'll see, time will tell. I know and trust that when the time is right, a man will be a significant part of my life.

MARCH 9

I almost didn't write today. It's practically midnight, and I was heading to bed when I realized I didn't prepare my hot water bottle. It's necessary at this time of year, so I figured I'll take the opportunity to write while the water's heating up. It's fascinating how easy it is to not keep my commitments to myself. I wonder why that is?

I had a good day. Yoga class was lovely; I had a pretty good turnout and a few people committed to the whole series. I went to the market, got my locally raised lamb and arranged a soil source for my secret garden. Got some good hugs in and a lovely conversation about how sweet it is to live in a community "where everyone knows my name," taking the quote from the TV show, *Cheers*.

My energy began to wane in the afternoon. I went for a Breema session with my friend, Claudia. It was lovely, very gentle and soothing and, by the end of it, I was so relaxed that I barely wanted to move. I dragged my butt home and crawled into bed for what was supposed to be a 30-minute power nap and didn't get out of bed until two hours later. I probably would have stayed in bed all night if it wasn't for my friend's birthday party. I'm glad I went as it was a wonderful gathering of souls. Good food, live music, lots of kids, even a baby that I got to hold for a precious time. Oh, that yearning to be a mother. I wonder if that dream will come true. Someone at the party was saying she didn't want to try having children at age forty-three because of the risk of Down syndrome. I didn't know that was a risk. That's about what age I'll be if it happens. I trust it will all work out. I'm healthy and strong. I've taken great care of my body and my health. What will be will be.

Going back to the party, I noticed that I'm getting to feel more at ease with people, or at least when I noticed that I was feeling shy or unsure of myself, I just reminded myself to breath and be present. No need to impress or prove myself. At one point I did go out and hang with the dog for a bit. I oddly feel more comfortable with animals than I do with other humans most of the time. I guess it comes from growing up an only child with two dogs and three cats. My pets were my best friends and siblings. Of course I do enjoy the company of people; in fact, I crave it and am learning how to be myself and more at ease with others. I had an insight last spring during my dark period that I'll share with you some time. It's about belonging.

I need to get to bed right now. It's late and I have to get up early for my radio show. I've chosen all the songs I want to play, but I don't feel like I want to say much tomorrow. I'm dedicating it to the memory of the boy who died tragically last Saturday. I wasn't sure if it was appropriate as the accident was a week ago already, and I thought people might want to move on, but I saw that his memorial is tomorrow right after my show, so it's actually perfect. I didn't know him or his family, but I still feel the loss and the impact on the community so I'd like to pay my respects and offer my support in this way.

I feel like I need to sit down and do a full-on writing session, for a few hours or so. So much has been going on for me that I want to capture and share. Plus, I think with the longer writing sessions, more depth will come through rather than this continual skimming of the surface. I'll try to do that this weekend and to prioritize time for ongoing writing sessions that are longer. Time slips away amazingly fast. I don't want the years to slip away without finishing this book. I must reaffirm my commitment and keep making it a priority. So be it. Good night.

MARCH 10

A fascinating day. I feel oddly both at peace and unsettled at the same time. I guess that's how I often feel: not quite fully at peace and not quite in a frenzy. Somewhere in between, surfing between the worlds—chaos and order, earth and spirit, mind and heart— although I learnt something last summer that profoundly shifted my perspective of the mind and its function. In Chinese, the symbol for heart is the same as for mind; they are one in the same.

Wow, the wind is picking up again. It's whistling through the trees. The weather, as it often does, is reflecting my inner world. This morning it was grey and overcast. After yoga, at about noon, the sun came out for a while and then it became cloudy again, with a few spatterings of rain and a gusting wind. A mixed bag of emotions and feelings swirling around. I was down at the beach gathering mussels and oysters with some friends and was struck by the sheer beauty and wonder of this land. How amazing that I get to live in such a beautiful place and enjoy the abundance of the sea. It was my first time harvesting wild mussels. I look forward to the delicious feast that my friends are preparing for tonight. Sometimes it's actually hard to accept how amazing my life is, how blessed I am. Especially when so many people in the world are suffering or struggling. And yet, compared to some others, I hardly have anything of 'value,' no prized possessions. All of the value in my life comes from nature and the people I am blessed to share my life with. My life is definitely about quality versus quantity.

After watching *Sacred Economics* the other day, I had a familiar impulse that I've had off and on throughout the years, to drop out of the economic money game altogether and just simply offer what I have to share for the pure joy of it. That feels like the more generous and trusting way to be, especially since I don't enjoy or agree with the whole economic system and money game. But then I think, "I do have rent to pay and I do enjoy things that money buys." So I do need to play the game. I wish I could find a way to do both. I do in a way; I trade my services for others' goods and services. I haven't done it in an outward and active way.

I would love to try an experiment and, for a month or two, just offer my services to anyone who wants or needs them, and people can give back whatever they want. Just to see what happens. Maybe I'll do that for the next five weeks that I am here, before I leave for Israel. Just for the fun of it and to see what happens. I can post a list of goods and services I need, or not. Just leave it open ended. I have almost enough money to get me through to May (I ended up getting a tax refund that was exactly what I needed to live on until my job at Hollyhock starts up again). If I have to take a little more from my credit, so be it. The idea excites me actually. It's something I've wanted to do for a long time but didn't have the courage or gumption to try it. There's nothing to lose. I feel it could be quite liberating actually, to break out of the money game and then come back to it by choice. Clear some karma there and some belief systems. I feel this amazing energy welling up from inside of me, from my solar plexus up to my heart centre, and I feel an opening and sense of clarity in my skull and mind. When this happens, I know I'm onto something that is true and good for me. It feels like another piece of integrity that's been missing. Trying to play by somebody else's rules, trying to fit into this system that I don't understand or agree with. I'm excited and fascinated to see what opens up from it. I love life experiments, especially ones where I get to break out of a box, imposed or self-generated.

I'm reminded of a book I was reading once, *Busting Loose from the Money Game*. I was trying to do an experiment back then. Actually, it was almost a year ago exactly, but that's when I began to have my breakdown and, again, I felt like I was trying to break free by somebody else's system or rules. The 'busting loose' approach wasn't clicking or making sense to me back then. So, yes, listening to and trusting my own inner guidance system is one of my practices in building confidence and faith in myself. Even if my experiment doesn't work, the act of following my own intuitions and heart's calling is what matters. It's not about the outcome, whether I win or lose, it's about how I play the game.

Do you ever feel pulled in two different directions or feel like you're caught between two worlds? I do—constantly. At one point I realized that it may have something to do with one side of my family being Jewish and the other German. The conflict began in my genes; it's in my cells and lives itself out in my psyche and life. I am a walking and breathing paradox, and perhaps part of my life's mission is to resolve that paradox, to bridge these two worlds. I have no idea how to do it or if it's even possible. But hey, I believe in a paradigm in which everything is possible so why not go for it.

The conflict I am facing now, the way it's playing out, is between the pursuit of knowing one's Self and the yogic view that there is no self to be known. Here I am developing a program for youth, centred around the importance of knowing who you are and knowing what's important to create a life of meaning and fulfillment. And then Stephen Cope is saying it's pointless, it's impossible to truly know who we are. We are unknowable, which I actually get on some level—it makes perfect sense. To say I know who I am would put limitations on myself, and ultimately there are none. I am infinite potential and possibility; yet this life is so geared around creating myself as 'someone' and around discovering my unique gifts—what it is that I am here for, what it is that will fulfill my purpose. It's all crazy making. What's it all for?

One moment I'm drawn to make the most of my life, cherish the time that I have, especially with the people that are important to me. At another point in time, I am discovering that it's all an illusion and all pointless and that any effort or energy put into this life actually creates suffering because I would be feeding a false identity that will eventually crumble and fall away. No attachments.

And yet Charles Eisenstein is saying that we need each other to create meaning and intimacy in our lives, that our life's purpose is to love and be loved, and that we are here to be of service to each other. Yet we are supposedly all one and return to the same cosmic soup where we all came from and, therefore, it doesn't matter. Yet we create karma if we do bad or harm and, hence, we have to keep working through our stuff, to learn that we are the cause of our lives and to experience the effects of our choices and actions. And yet we ultimately don't have choice; our destiny is already determined and surrender is the highest and only true way. It's quite hilarious actually.

So what does it all mean? What's the point of it all? What do I take from this? To just live my life day by day, follow my heart, honour my own truth, live my life in integrity with what rings true for me moment to moment and allow my truth to change. To not take anything too seriously, be the best person I can be, make the most of my life and try to have as much enjoyment in the process as possible without doing harm to anyone or anything so that I can be at peace within myself and sleep at night with a clear conscience.

But hey, maybe that's the wimpy way out, maybe the boldest way to live would be to take as many risks as possible; don't give a shit about what anyone thinks; see how much destruction I can make; break free from all rules, laws and judgments; be a bad ass; and create havoc. Who's to say one is any better than the other. It's all perspective right?! Quite fascinating really. If we truly are here as a game to experience what it is to be human, to have the full human experience, why should being an upstanding Samaritan be any better than a mass murderer? It's all great and fun brain candy, but ultimately I'm not willing to take that risk. There is some deep calling in me to keep expanding my capacity to love and connect, to honour and cherish all life and so that is my chosen path. Perhaps someday it will change, but for now I will honour and trust that call. Some good late night philosophizing.

MARCH 11

I had a fleeting moment this morning at Kirtan when it all made perfect sense. I totally understood the paradox, the masculine (nothingness, space, consciousness) and the feminine (form, expression, creation) aspects that make up the whole. I could see how it was all God, but then my mind went to murdering someone, and I couldn't find God in that somehow, even though a part of me suspects that it is, but I'm not convinced.

Shoot, it was a gorgeous sunny day and now the grey clouds are moving in, and I haven't been out for my walk yet. I needed to eat and was just having some tea when I decided to capture some of my thoughts from this morning. I also wanted to account a dream I had last night. One aspect of it stuck very clearly; I was in some meeting, an evaluation of my performance at 'work' as some speaker or pre-senter, and a woman—who might have been my supervisor—told me, "Use less words, say less," basically, "Get to the point." I wonder if that's my subconscious trying to tell me that I'm being a little too verbose in my writing and should try to get to the essence or 'heart' of what I'm trying to say. I'll work on that. ;-)

The sun is gone. It's windy. I'm done my tea, but now I just want to sleep rather than go for a walk. Fascinating. I wonder why I'm so tired lately. I've been getting nine hours of sleep most nights, but it doesn't seem to be enough. I have been quite active and busy. I have to remember the balance between being active and engaged and taking time for myself to be still and quiet. It's silly though because as I write that, I think about being a parent and how indulgent getting lots of sleep and personal time is. Maybe that's why it's so important to me now, to get it while I can. I still wonder whether I will have the opportunity to give birth. I really do hope so but I'm lacking the certainty. So many factors involved, a man being a big one. ;-) That makes me chuckle. I'm not sure why—I guess the absurdity of it.

Then of course, there's the finances. But as I write this, I think of how many women are out there that have had children without worrying about these things. They just did it. Maybe because my childhood was so unsettling with both of my parents not totally being there for me and not having much money that it's become imperative to give the things that I didn't receive to my own child or children.

Wow, it's become really stormy out there now. What a switch— from sunny and gorgeous to grey and blustery. The weather never ceases to amaze me. And yes, I am talking about the weather. Oh my God, it just started hailing now! Wild!! I guess it's a good thing that I wasn't out there walking. I'd be caught in a hail storm right now. It's pounding down hard! I wonder how many people are caught in this on a beach somewhere. Crazy, intense and beautiful at the same time. Ooh, a sun shower now! That's my absolute favourite, when the sun and the rain happen at the same time. Quite magical. Now there's just a mist of rain in the air, and the sun is radiating through and creating a shimmery shine to the air. The time is13:33, on 11/03/2012. Sometimes numbers fascinate me. Threes and eights have a special meaning for me. Eight is my symbol in the Mayan Astrology; 3s I'm not even sure why. I lived at 333-E13 once. Age thirty-three was a powerful year for me. I think the Buddha and Christ had their moments of awakening at age thirty-three.

I can't stop eating chocolate. I guess I just shouldn't have any in the house. I'd probably just walk to the store and get some then. I'm rambling and talking in circles again. Get to the point! What is the point? In essence I'm feeling kind of lonely, and I think I'm trying to avoid that. Perhaps even deny it. Trying to be strong. I'm supposed to be okay with myself and not need anyone, but I do. Yes, there's the sadness now. It's been named and acknowledged. I've been trying to override it, keep busy so I can't/won't feel it. But it's always there, just under the surface, no matter how busy I am, how much I do. I yearn to be with another, to share my life with someone. I have a really amazing life. I am quite in awe of it actually. I was feeling the awe this morning while at Kirtan and even just sitting here in my beautiful home surrounded by my musical instruments, my art, plants, trees, birds. I have most everything I could ever want except that ever elusive beloved. And yes, as I write that, I know the beloved is everywhere, in everyone, and I share my love and my heart with many, but it's not the same, at least not to me at this point in my life. My heart is awakened now, I can feel it, I literally feel sensation there. I can't quite place what it is—an ache? An opening? A stirring? It's difficult to name, but I feel it—the sadness, tears just below the surface, welling up, an expression of the sadness but also tears of relief. The relief of being acknowledged and known. The relief and tears of acceptance. A big sigh now, a settling in to myself, the restlessness and fatigue dissipating into the space of okayness.

The sun is streaming through my window now, almost in celebration of this subtle shift into what is true. So simple and so sweet, even in its exquisite pain, because it is real, it is what's so. A softening, even a tangible presence of grace. I see how I've been trying so hard, to earn, to win, to attract, to do whatever I can to 'make it happen' when really what was needed was to stop, breathe, feel and allow. Funny, it comes back to needing to learn what I teach. Of course. The sun beckons me now, into the great blue yonder I go.

FACEBOOK STATUS/BLOG ENTRY:

As of this moment until midnight on April 13, 2012, I am embarking on a journey into new territory, exploring life outside the limitations of the money-based economic system. I am busting loose from the money game. As an act of faith, guided by my heart, inspired by *Sacred Economics* and the Occupy movement, I offer my love, my energy and my services as a gift to whoever is in need of or requests my presence and/or assistance. I reserve the right to say no. I will still use money as an energy exchange but am not limited to it. I expect nothing in return and will accept all offerings (goods, services, praise, money, etc.). This is an experiment to see what happens, to break free of old and limiting beliefs, to be in full integrity with what I value in my heart to be true, to be a pure and generous source of love and contribution to my community and society. Am I scared? Hell ya! Am I excited? You bet! Anyone care to join me on this wild and wacky ride? I welcome reflections, feedback and encouragement.

MARCH 12

Hollywood has spoiled me, has ruined all of my chances at experiencing real love. I am too caught up in the fantasy of relationship and romance as portrayed in the movies. I feel hopeless. I wonder what I am doing wrong, or how I could be different. They say if you don't like the outcome of your actions then you must change your actions. Or rather, something about results staying the same ... oh, I can't remember. It's something Theda told me once. Don't expect different results if you don't change what you're doing. I suck at remembering sayings and quotes and such.

**Insanity is doing the same thing over and over again
and expecting different results.
~ Albert Einstein**

I do feel stuck somehow. In the area of romance and relationship. Even though I am kind of dating someone and just had a torrid love affair with a beautiful man. Something still isn't quite clicking. I feel like I'm missing something about me, my internal workings, some mechanism inside me that is preventing true fulfillment in this area. Perhaps I have some unconscious belief or fear or protective mechanism/shell. I don't know obviously; otherwise, if I did know, then I would perhaps be able to do something about it. I feel somewhat broken inside, some piece or aspect of my being that is missing that could open me up to and allow a real and true lasting relationship into my life. What is it? It's so frustrating. The thing that I yearn for most in my life, and it completely eludes me.

I see all these people in real life and in movies who are not perfect—flawed—and they end up falling in love and sharing their

From My
Heart
To Yours

life with someone. Why not me? What am I missing? Some big life lesson? Oh, God, please don't let me be destined to be alone. Maybe that's it—I have to work through and abandon this fear of being alone before I earn the right to be with another. Seems ridiculous and unfair. But hey, that's definitely one of my limiting beliefs that I'm aware of, "Life is unfair." And I know that life is neither fair nor unfair or rather is both.

Sadness is welling up again, tears of despair, heartbreak. Sometimes I feel so self-absorbed. Why can't I just live my life, this truly amazing and blessed life that I have the privilege to have? So many blessings, and yet all seem so empty without someone to share them with.

I've been obsessing over this man who I had an encounter with last weekend. I went into it knowing it was a one-time fling, but now I'm not so sure. Or at least fantasizing that it could be more. It was such a powerful and unexpected encounter. Passionate, hot, sexy, fun and yet also enchanting. I can't remember if I described it or not.

I was at a contact dance event. I almost didn't go because I was feeling tired and uninspired and was wishing I was back on Cortes. My friends who I was going to go with had both fallen asleep, and so I was left with the option of joining them or going on my own. I had decided to meditate and then probably go to bed, but some internal voice kept nagging at me. I still wasn't convinced so I decided to do the trusty muscle test. I made an O with my left thumb and forefinger and put my right thumb and forefinger inside the circle. If when I tug the left circle holds, it's a yes; if the ring breaks, it's a no. When I asked myself, "Is it in my highest good and in the highest good of all for me to go to contact dance?" The circle held strong, so I threw on a pair of loose comfortable pants and a comfy shirt. Thought nothing of 'making myself presentable or beautiful' and headed out.

I got there late. The 'journey' had already started so I slipped in, found a space on the floor and began to let my body move to the music. Someone I knew and had danced with in contact dance classes and jams was guiding the room. I guess she had already led them through a warm-up because, a few minutes after I arrived, she was guiding people to partner up and explore the dance of connection. My first dance was with a lovely young woman. A bit tentative and shy, we explored the dance of our hands in contact with each other. Eventually we allowed the dance to move down our arms and, at some point, down our bodies. It was sweet, playful and lighthearted.

I felt the stiffness in my body begin to melt away and a giddiness began to emerge.

The next couple of dances were with men who obviously had never contact danced before and were there to get their rocks off. I kept the contact light and playful and found humour in the whole situation. I found myself laughing in delighted amusement often.

One of my favourite moments from the evening was when she had us all go to one end of the room and begin to roll like waves over to the other side. Legs, arms, torsos all colliding and rolling over each other, sometimes a whole body surfing up and over the giant wave that we had become as a whole. It was hilarious. We ended up in a heap of laughter in front of the DJ booth. People peeling off the big puddle of mush we had created, like drops evaporating off the ocean. Duets and trios began to fill the dance floor once again.

When I made my way to standing to join the dance, I ended up being ricocheted from person to person like a ball in a pinball machine. It was quite fun. Then all of a sudden this masculine form broke off from a trio of men to join me in a dance that rocked my socks—well, would have if I'd been wearing any. At any rate, it was hot, a little too hot, and I was feeling uncomfortable so I politely broke away from the dance feigning thirst. He bowed and said, "Arigato" then twirled away to join the duet of elderly men once again. I went and got my drink of water and caught my breath. I thought, "That was fun" and left it at that.

I felt the need to do some solo dancing so I twirled around the floor for a while, giving myself over to the music when all of a sudden a body was against mine once again. It was him! He was back. At first I was at odds as to what to do, but the dance has a life of its own so I gave over to it. I was caught in its/his web. I'm a sucker for a great dance(r). Before I know it, the music has stopped, and I'm on the floor belly down or in child's pose—I can't quite remember. But I do distinctly remember his body on mine, his face nuzzled into the back of my neck, his hot breath, his sensual caress, our deep and heavy breathing in unison. It felt like he had been making love to me on the dance floor. I was intoxicated, caught in some spell. We lay there for what seemed like hours. Finally I needed to shift my body, I think my arm was falling asleep or something silly like that. I rolled over onto my back and into his arms, looked up into his face and in a daze, and gasped, "Who are you?"

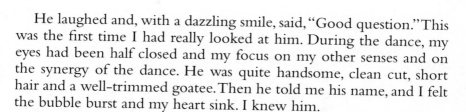

He laughed and, with a dazzling smile, said, "Good question." This was the first time I had really looked at him. During the dance, my eyes had been half closed and my focus on my other senses and on the synergy of the dance. He was quite handsome, clean cut, short hair and a well-trimmed goatee. Then he told me his name, and I felt the bubble burst and my heart sink. I knew him.

One of my best girlfriend's had had a fling with him. In fact, the friend that was supposed to be with me that evening but had instead stayed in the cozy warmth of her bed. She had really liked him, and yet she now has a boyfriend. I felt confused and torn. And couldn't help but laugh at the absurdity of it all. I exclaimed in my laughter, "How hilarious life is." I told him we knew each other. He assured me that he would have remembered meeting me. Very smooth and sweet. I told him that it had been a long time ago and that he had dated one of my best girlfriends.

Recognition clicks and he said, "Well, that could only be one person." It doesn't seem to faze him. He asks if I'm hungry. He's definitely made up his mind and nothing will deter him. I tell him no, but I would love some tea.

To make a long story short, we end up at his place. He makes me tea and shows me his place, which is a bit disastrous. He just returned from a trip to Costa Rica, but I have a feeling it's just an excuse. He's an artist, large canvases, paint, big chunks of wood, clothing, artifacts and children's toys (he has a 3-year-old son) are scattered through his modest basement suite. He's also a carpenter, builds houses, owns a boat, loves travel and adventure. I'm enamoured. He's a great storyteller, too. He pours the tea and smoothly beckons me into his bedroom.

I'm still not sure of what to do at this point. I tell myself, "Tea is harmless." Still torn about the duties of a friend versus the charms of a sexy, attentive and seductive man. He gets me with the coconut oil massage and the biting of my neck. Oh, yes, there's the promise of blueberry pancakes in the morning. He's very good. Still a little guarded and unsure, I slowly succumb as he melts each layer of resistance with a kiss, a caress, a praise, a tousle. I'm a total sucker for male attention, sensuality and seduction.

Well, let me qualify something. I don't just give in to any type of male attention. Just that of a certain quality. He certainly met my criteria. He was sweet, generous, present, funny, handsome, witty, sensual and attentive, and he had that certain quality that particularly seductive men have—that touch of danger, roughness. It's almost indescribable. His touch was that perfect mix of firmness and tenderness. Yep, he got me, got me good. But my mind still wasn't convinced. I staved him off for quite a while, but he was very convincing. I don't know if it was because my mind hadn't let me be fully receptive or open to the experience, but when we finally did make love, it was kind of disappointing. He came quickly and before me. I told him, in a playful joking way, "You know that a gentleman brings the woman to pleasure first" and he came back with, "Well, I never said I was a gentleman, did I?" and makes his way down to ... (It's very difficult to write about this. It would be one thing if I was telling a story, but this is me and my life that I'm sharing with God knows whoever will read this, so I'm going to fast forward a little—probably to your dismay—sorry ;-).

So, anyway, let's just say that luckily for him—and for me—he made a very quick recovery. We made love three more times. I was impressed and grateful to finally be with a man with a good and healthy libido. True to his word, he made me blueberry pancakes for breakfast, and we ended our encounter with a lovely walk along the beach. Walking arm in arm or hand in hand and feeling quite comfortable with each other, we shared stories of our lives. I dropped him off at his truck, he gave me his card and a kiss and told me to call him sometime if I ever come back to the city or perhaps he'd find his way to my island. That was just over a week ago, I haven't called him, and I still don't know if I should.

Part of me just wants to let it go and not get caught up in his charm, and the other part of me wonders if there is some possibility there, some potential ... for what? I don't know. I'm letting my friend's experience with him influence my judgment, which may be good or not. But I also feel I'm letting fear and pettiness get in the way of ... of what? Again, I'm not sure. But I will never know unless I give it a chance, right? What do I have to lose, some pride. I'm going to go for a walk. I'll know when and if I'm ready to call. Or maybe my friend, Theda, is right. Maybe with certain choices, one is never ready, and you just have to take that leap. I'll decide when I get back from my walk.

I want to write, but my battery is running out, and our power is out from the storm and not due to come back on until tomorrow evening sometime. I'll write until I can't. I'm going through something strange. All I want to do is eat; I'm obviously trying to stuff something. Not wanting to feel, avoiding the pangs of loneliness. Why is it that when I don't have the attention of some man, rather than spend my time doing good for myself, I fall to bad habits that aren't good for my health or well-being?

I decided not to call Tony (that's what we'll call the city man—the enchanter). I don't want to make a call to him out of desperation, which is how I am feeling right now. I will perhaps call him sometime when I am feeling clear and empowered. Is that my defense mechanism coming up now, not wanting to be vulnerable? Argh, I'm such a complex being, or perhaps I'm actually quite simple, and I just make myself out to be complicated. If that makes any sense.

Anyway, I had a lovely walk through the woods down to the maple tree, which is a special spot on the ocean. I sat, walked and lay in the sun for hours. It was beautiful, eagles soared overhead, a heron landed nearby, the sun was warm and the sound of the ocean soothing. Yet I still couldn't shake that feeling of discontent. I wondered if it was my 'Enneagram' imprinting. According to my friend, I'm a seven in the Enneagram, and we are chronically discontented and seeking the next thrill. This is an ongoing theme in my life for sure. *I have since discovered that I am actually a four in the Enneagram, which is described as being a moody dreamer and hopeless romantic in search of true love. Definitely fitting. ;-) Like all systems, these tools are available for guidance and assistance but not to be taken as absolute truth. I believe that the truth of who we are is beyond all systems.*

ENNEAGRAM

The Enneagram is a model of human personality, which is principally used as a typology of nine interconnected personality types. Principally developed by Oscar Ichazo and Claudio Naranjo, it is also partly based on earlier teachings of G. I. Gurdjieff. In spirituality, it is commonly presented as a path to higher states of being, essence and enlightenment. It has been described as a method for self-understanding and self-development. ~ Wikipedia

I also remember having a fascinating thought while I was walking through the woods, which was that I seem to need my value affirmed by either receiving money or male attention. If I'm not getting either, I don't feel valuable. I feel worthless or unimportant somehow. Like I need either money or men to feel validated. Yeah, I feel I'm on to something because those are the two ongoing biggest challenges I face in life: money and men.

Some of you are probably saying, "Yeah, so? You and most other women on this planet." Or do they? Probably. Fascinating. I don't mean to come across as a manhater or anything but wasn't it men who created money? Don't get me wrong; I love men, crazy about them in fact, more like obsessed over them. And I know many men who are as unhappy with the economic system as I am. In fact, it was three men who inspired me to do the experiment I'm doing right now around money: Velcrow Ripper, Ian Mackenzie and Charles Eisenstein. I need/want a man like that in my life, someone who is doing something meaningful with their life for a cause that I totally believe in. I want to share and co-create my life with someone who shares the same values, visions, passions and dreams. Someone to create magic with, to experience the magic that life has to offer. To weather the storms with, to explore new territory with, to laugh, cry, sing, dance and make love with. Oh yeah, I remember another thought that arose during my walk, something about not feeling worthy or deserving of a partner. Where does this shit come from? Why would I deny myself that which I most desire?

Oh yeah, and then I had the thought that perhaps I do need to learn a lesson first, I need to learn to be happy and content in myself before I can be with another. But, come on! What if that's a 'mission impossible'?! I know tons of people who are in relationship and who haven't achieved full self-fulfillment and self-realization. What if that's the limiting belief that's getting in my way, that perfectionist part of me that feels I need to have it all together first? Maybe!

I just had the thought that nobody should need to have to 'earn' love. I don't need to prove myself to deserve to be loved. That's proof right there that the thought, "I need to learn a lesson first" is false. I definitely call bullshit on that one. I am deserving of love right now, just as I am. Yeah, that's a big one. Good to expose that puppy. I am love-able! I deserve love just as I am, I am worthy of love. I love to give and to receive love. I was born to love! I am love! Please, God, let this stick this time. I open the floodgates of my heart to give and receive love, endlessly, without limit. My purpose on this planet, in this life, is to love. I am a lover. I live to love to live. That's my motto, time to live up to it. Walk my talk. Okay, stop being hard on yourself, Shaeah. You have been doing that; you are just reaching another level, breaking through a little dam that was created around your heart. Remember the journey is about ever expanding my capacity to love. It's a journey, not a competition. Just keep doing your best. Trust yourself, trust in life, trust in 'God/ Spirit/ the Divine/ the Universe'—what have you.

This reminds me of something else that came to me while I was at the beach—that I need to remember to trust and have faith. I know when I get too much in my head, I start to doubt and question my life, and that's when I need to remember to come back to my heart and trust. And then as I say that, I am remembering that the heart and the mind are supposedly one and the same. If so, then why are they so often (or at least seem to be) in conflict with each other? Another one of life's mysteries. With that, I'll bid you adieu and good night.

March 14

Vancouver Island

Another storm is brewing; it's 4:30am and I can't sleep. I'm at my newish friends' place on Vancouver Island. I came over yesterday for an appointment and decided to stay over for a few reasons. One, I had no power at home. Two, I needed to take my car into be serviced, and three, I really like this couple and wanted to spend more time getting to know them.

There's something about them that is quite magnetic. I find them quite magical actually, and I don't think they even know how magical they are. That's part of their charm—how humble and modest they both are. They live in a beautiful storybook home they built about eleven years ago. They are both creative geniuses and, like I said, they don't even know it or maybe they do and they …no, I don't think they truly know how brilliant they are. Her art, inspired by Dr. Seuss, is bright bold and delightful to behold. She's a painter amongst many other things, of course. She's kind of like me that way. She even said today, while we were driving in the car back to their place, that she can't just pursue one job or interest or she gets bored. I feel exactly the same way.

Even though we seem quite different on the outside, I feel very much like we are kindred spirits at heart. I was enamoured with her the first time I saw her at the SARK workshop, which is where I met them. Her first, him later (he wasn't in the workshop, but was just there for the time away and to support her—he's very lovely that way, supportive that is). They were teenage sweethearts, fell in love, got married and have been together ever since. Almost unheard of at this day and age. He's an inventor type. He is interested in sustainability and alternative energy. His heart oozes from his gentle nature. I don't feel like I'm capturing them well enough. I'm not sure if it's the fatigue or the sheer incapability of portraying who they are in writing. Too limiting. I feel like they could do anything as they are powerful creative brilliant manifesters with the most incredibly generous and loving spirits. Even their names are magical: Naomi and Nico teWinkle. I'm obviously enchanted and inspired by who they are.

The first time I really got to know them was playing the Transformation Game with them at Hollyhock. It's a four-player game, but we did it with five. The two of them paired up and it worked perfectly. That's how connected they are. They were talking tonight about how they had read somewhere that couples after a while stop using the parts of their brain that the other person is stronger/better at. As a unit, they are a complete brain, but on their own each has lost certain functions. She has lost the ability to make oatmeal in the mornings; I forget what he has lost the ability to do. It was quite sweet how they talked about it. They are very playful. We laughed a lot as we played SARK's Creative Dream game last night and watched a great romantic comedy: *Crazy, Stupid, Love.*

My creative dream that I focussed on was this book. The learning that I took away from the game was to ask for and receive more help and support. As I was lying awake listening to the sound of the wind through the trees and the tinkling of the chimes, I decided that I'm going to ask for someone to help me edit my book. During the game, I decided that I was just going to give a few pages to one or two people to read and get their feedback—which I'll still probably do—but I see that getting an editor is a more committed and solid step to making this book happen. I'm also to sketch the cover to make it more concrete; that was a micro-movement (small steps towards my goal/dream) that came to me. Oh yeah, I was gifted the 'cloak of patience' for those times when I feel the book should already be done or it should be progressing faster. I need to remember to enjoy the process rather than to concentrate solely on the goal of finishing the book—as I look down to see what page number I'm at! ;-) So typical. At least I can have humour with myself.

I'm to be aware of my resistance, which has been manifesting as waiting until the last possible moment to write, when I'm tired and feel it as a chore rather than a pleasure. So, I've decided to make a more concerted effort to go for a walk in the morning and to write when I get back from my walk when I'm feeling clear and inspired.

Shaeah Love : **79**

Oh yeah, there was something about energy. What gives me more expanded energy? Do more of that. Walking and being in nature, dancing, getting massages and spending quality time with friends and family. I have notes on all of the insights, which I received during the game, written on a piece of paper, but I'm sitting in the dark and don't feel like turning on any lights to look for it so I'm just going by memory.

Oh yeah, I remember one fun one. I think it was a 'Gift' card, and it said, "Lie down immediately," so I did. I went to lie down on the floor in front of the fireplace where Charlie, the ginger kitty, was curled up on his sheepskin. He was startled and moved away so I was able to actually lie down on his lovely warm spot. The message I received while lying there was to make sure I get enough rest so that I am able and available to allow the creativity to flow through me more easily. I think I'm good at getting lots of rest, but the piece that I got from that card is to let it be okay. Sometimes I get down on myself for needing to sleep or rest so much. I make it wrong and mean that I'm lazy. Rest is supportive and necessary for the creative process, she says at 5:10am. Sometimes you just got to flow with it, when the energy and creative juices are flowing, go with it. Ebb and flow! Trust the process.

I'm starting to yawn. Feels like almost time to go back to bed. But I want to capture a few inspirations first. While I was lying in bed wide awake, I got the idea to focus my coaching and Clearing support to help people realize their creative dreams. Help people with specific projects that inspire them and help fulfill a dream of theirs. I'm going to start by offering support to my two magical friends to help them realize the creative dreams they worked on last night in our game. Whoa, run-on sentence. Yep, I need an editor! ;-)

Another inspiration I've had is to write a little book about *Money, Men and Magic*. I don't know what it will say exactly, but it's super catchy and keeps getting stronger in my head. It could be another one of those passing fancies but, on the other hand, I could be on to something.

Oh yeah, that was another message from the game last night: 'mistakes.' I think it was permission to make mistakes. What 'mistakes' can I learn from in past creative endeavours? One is that I have a habit of giving up on myself and my projects. So I have reaffirmed my commitment to this one. I need to get myself a coach/mentor for this project. Oh yeah, that was the first card I pulled under the 'Love' topic. Allies, mentors, teachers. I need to find new ones because I seem to have outgrown or let go of my past ones. Or I could just reconnect with some of them. I have had the impulse to call my friend Stephen lately. *He's a past colleague and mentor that has written a couple of books.* That's a great idea. But I also feel the pull to find some new sources of mentorship. It'd be great to find a woman who has written a book. Order up! That's my call out to the Universe. We'll see how and where she shows up. I'll keep you posted. I think that's all I have to share right now.

Hey, I just want to say, thanks for listening, or reading. I feel like you're listening. You're hearing my voice through the pages or maybe literally if this has become an audio book! Now that's a fun thought.

Life is great, isn't it?! Quite a hoot. I hope you're enjoying it, if not do something about it. Seriously, it's in your hands. Life's too short to mess around unless you really want to, but know that suffering is optional—certain forms of it anyway. You have the ability to make certain choices that can transform your experience of life. I know because I've done it over and over again. Part of my intention for this book is to turn my story into a rags-to-riches one, to inspire you, to prove that it's possible not only to you but to myself. And you know I may not strike it rich but, in the process of trying, I'm transforming my experience of life into a richer one. That's all that matters. It's inspiring me to share myself more fully, to find my voice, to find humour and enjoyment in my life, to connect more deeply and openly to myself and with others. That is success and fulfillment to me. The money would be great, too; I'm not so sure about the fame anymore, but I'll take whatever's meant to come. I'm learning to trust myself and life more and more and that feels great. I guess that's what they call faith.

FACEBOOK STATUS/BLOG ENTRY:

Day three. I'm stuck on Vancouver Island due to the ferries not running. Luckily I have the generous and warm hospitality of some dear friends. I'm experiencing the paradox of life, feeling the sweetness of good-hearted people and enjoying their company, and I'm happy to spend more time with them. But I'm facing the disappointment of having to miss the yoga class that I teach, letting students down and feeling stressed about the money I'm losing from that. To add salt to the wound, I had to turn down some other paid work that came up. This was compounded by the $350 mechanics bill. I definitely had my money buttons pushed today. I noticed the stress I was feeling as I drove to my friends' from the mechanics, knowing I was missing my yoga class and paid work. Not a great feeling to feel stress of money overtake my faith.

But I take it as a great opportunity to see those unconscious beliefs get flushed out. The key is to not take it as truth. One of the main intentions of this journey is to break free of these limiting beliefs and the first step in that is bringing them to consciousness. This is the icky part of the process, where I have to feel the yuck of these beliefs. It's difficult to share about this part because I want to be seen as already free and generous. But I am committed to being totally transparent during this process, both to provide learning and inspiration to whoever reads this and for my own benefit (being witnessed adds power to any process). I've settled into and accepted where I'm at. I'll keep you posted.

I Am A Lover!!!
Cortes Island

The economist says, 'the more I give the less I have,'
the lover says, 'the more I give the more I have.'
~ Charles Eisenstein, *Sacred Economics*

I'm back home, cozied in my bed listening to the blustering winds get stronger again. But at least they cleared long enough to let me get home. I just caught the window when the ferries could run. I have just reread my blogs on my website, from September 2009 on. Wow, they're good. I was inspired by my own writing. Makes me wish I had kept it up more. There are so many gaps. Oh well, gives me more impetus to keep writing this book. I have a voice with powerful and meaningful things to say that will hopefully have an impact and inspire others. That would be you. Doesn't it bother you when people talk about you in third person, especially when you're right there? As I read my earlier writing, I actually feel like I had more insight back then. I guess that's my critic coming in. I don't know, maybe I was just more idealistic and now I'm more realistic—but hopefully both. Not too much or too little of one or the other, but a good balance would be the ideal. Ha, there I go being the idealist! Hee hee.

It is a fascinating time for me. I feel like I am finally stepping out more fully and sharing myself in a way I have always envisioned or hoped but was too insecure or shy or simply not ready for. And that's okay. I just watched a preview for the movie *Milk* about Harvey Milk, and a line from there struck me, as I could perfectly relate to it: "I'm forty years old and what do I have to show for it? Nothing."

Then he goes on to make history (as a pioneer for gay rights), not to say that I will (make history, that is), but it's just nice to have affirmation that some of us are late bloomers.

From My
Heart
To Yours

MARCH 15

What a great day! It had such a beautiful flow to it. I started the day with Yoga Nidra and breakfast. Caught a window of sunshine for my bike ride to the hall for Qi Gong. Had an interview for the Adventures in Leadership Coordinator position and came away feeling really good about it. I was at ease, authentic and engaging, and I think I gave pretty intelligible answers to all of their questions. The greatest thing for me is that I felt I was able to be myself and, at the end, felt confident that I could do the job and actually would want to do the job. Going in I wasn't sure I really had what it takes. That's one of my ongoing limiting beliefs actually: "I don't have what it takes." Well, in this case, I think I do and, in fact, I think I would be really great at it and enjoy it.

On the way home I ran into someone who had contacted me about being my roommate, so I invited him over for tea. He loved the place, and we had a lovely visit. Sweet man. It's funny because I had put the posting out for a woman specifically, and my landlord and I had joked the other day, "Unless it's a very feminine man" and when this guy emailed me, he wrote, "Would you consider a very feminine man?" It gave me a giggle, and I took it as a sign to be open to the possibility. He's also writing a book and practices Vipassana. We'll see. There's a woman who's interested in coming on Saturday, and she contacted me first so, to be fair, I feel I should meet her and see if there's a match there.

After he left, I felt inspired to do some spring cleaning. I need to make space for my new roommate as I've spread out and taken over the place during the winter. I cranked the tunes and began clearing out all of the kitchen cupboards. I like cleaning. There's something very satisfying about it, probably because there's instant gratification in seeing the results immediately. I like order, too. I like the aesthetics of cups, glasses and plates lined up. I probably got it from my mom.

I certainly didn't get it from my dad. I'm really great at chaos, too, especially when I live on my own; there's something very satisfying about just letting things go and not being rigid. But I can only take it for so long and then I start to go a little crazy as it's difficult to focus in chaos. I find order and spaciousness allows for more freedom of expression and yet chaos is a form of freedom of expression. Fascinating, isn't it?! I love how contradictory life can be sometimes; at other times it drives me crazy. Anyway, I started to create some order in my kitchen but, if you were to look at it now, you would think it was in chaos. I got interrupted in the middle by a dear friend in need of some connection. Friends come first! Plus it was a good time for a break. We had tea, a snack and a good heart-to-heart talk.

Later we decided to go for a walk, on my favourite route; he was the one who had shown it to me. It was so amazing to get out. I hadn't realized until I was walking in the open air that I hadn't walked since Sunday. That's three days without my nature walk! My friend said he was glad that I had noticed that he didn't seem himself because he wasn't even aware that he had been withdrawn. I joked about drawing him out of his turtle shell. We skipped down the road arm in arm toward our trusty trail that ran past the lake to the waterfall. The waterfall was at its peak after all the storms. I could feel my cells coming more alive as I stood there absorbing all the negative ions. At one point, I shared with my friend that I had a crazy impulse to jump into the waterfall. It looked so inviting and enlivening. I resisted and we continued our walk to the lagoon. We stood on the sandy spit looking out at the snow-capped mountains, listening to the waves and the birds and feeling the wind caressing our faces. The scene felt dramatic and evoked something in me. I started singing a Madonna song, "Life is a Mystery" and went on to share my wish of being able to magically become an amazing musician who can break out into song.

I admire people who express themselves boldly and fully. Entertainers inspire me, I get such joy out of seeing people be wild and crazy on stage. I still aspire to be a great entertainer someday. Truly, if I wasn't contained and didn't hold myself back, that's what I would do. So what's stopping me? What's holding me back? Is it a true calling or just some childhood/adolescent fantasy? That voice again, "I don't have what it takes." Hmmm, interesting. It's still possible. I could become an amazing entertainer at any age or at any time I choose.

It's an exciting time in my life, not knowing what's ahead. I have been feeling a little pulled in opposite directions again though. One, the pull toward a dynamic exciting life of travel and adventure and the other toward setting up a nest and settling down. I don't know why my mind goes to either or. Do I have to choose? Or is it possible to have both?

My idealist says, "Oh yeah, of course, anything is possible."

My realist says, "I'm not so sure, you need to make some choices, honey."

I don't have to figure it out. I just have to keep following my heart and living with integrity, and it'll all work itself out. One step at a time. I sense that my choice of man will influence what's possible in my life.

And then the voice comes in, "You don't have a choice, honey. It's all decided, you just need to accept and allow what grace gives you."

But this sounds like settling to me. Argh, I'm back to that darn conundrum—life's major riddle. How much of my life is determined by my will and how much is determined by God/Spirit's will? Is there a difference? I ask myself as I recall the voice that came to me a few weeks back during my surrender yoga session, "My will is thy will." Again, I come back to, "If I follow my heart and live with integrity it will all sort itself out." Trust myself, trust the Universe, which are one in the same. So be it.

MARCH 16

**All alone! Whether you like it or not,
alone is something you'll be quite a lot!
~ Dr. Seuss, *Oh The Places You'll Go***

Something's troubling me. I can't sleep. It's half past midnight, and I've been lying in bed for over an hour, tossing and turning, a flood of thoughts flowing through my mind. I feel sad and a little lonely. It's crazy because my week has been so full with amazing connections and activities and with lots of great and lovely people but none of them romantic. That part of me is starving, aching, yearning to be fulfilled. And I don't know what to do about it. Except be with it. And that sucks. It feels really shitty and adolescent and unevolved. I feel captive to this emptiness, that there's no escape. I don't understand it, this feeling of discontent and despair when my life is so full and rich. What am I doing wrong? Am I destined to a life of loneliness and despair? Okay, now I'm being dramatic. That got a little chuckle out of me. And yet the heaviness of the heart remains. Maybe I'm starting to access some core belief, a big voice goes, "Duh! Do you think." Like it's blaringly obvious. I'm gathering it has something to do with being alone. I just wish I could get to the place where I was so fulfilled and happy within myself, and it didn't matter if I had a man to share it with. That's when they say it happens, when you don't need or want it to. And yet others say you need to feel the loneliness fully. I guess that's where I'm at 'cause I certainly ain't at the other place. I read a quote today that fits this scenario perfectly:

The curious paradox is that when I accept myself just as I am, then I can change. ~ Carl Rogers

Sometimes life pisses me off. With all its fucking paradox bullshit, this duality nonsense just doesn't make sense most of the time. Why do I have this ongoing feeling like I'm missing something, some significant secret key to finding true lasting love? If this kind of love didn't exist, so many songs wouldn't be written about it and so many movies wouldn't be made about it. Or are people doing that just to be cruel, to create this false sense or idea of what's possible. Is true everlasting love a fantasy? Faery tale? Hollywood?

I'm feeling that call to make a movie about love. I had an idea for. I wanted to go around and interview tons of people about love and get the real scoop on it, not just this Hollywood fantasy bullshit. What is it really? In real life, with real people? Why can it be so elusive at times and so enrapturing at other times?

Metaphysically, I need to look within myself and look at where I am not loving me. Of course, I always have room for improvement, but I think I'm doing my best. I eat really well—yes, I could eat better. I take good care of my body—yes, I could exercise more and do even more yoga. I do things that I love and enjoy—yes, I could play more music and dance even more. I am self-sufficient and take care of my basic needs—yes, I could improve in the area of financial and material wealth and well-being. I'm working on that one. Okay, self-acceptance and compassion are biggies.

But I feel I am more there than ever, and I know a lot of people who don't have those mastered, and they are in relationship. So what the fuck?! That fucking word, 'faith' comes up. Trust, surrender. What else can I do? I could call Tony, the city enchanter. I could reactivate my Plenty of Fish account. I could move somewhere where there are more men. No, then I'd be giving up the life I love for a man and that's not healthy. It comes back to trust and patience. Know that I am deserving of love and trust that it will come. In the meantime, focus on loving myself as best I can. And that includes this lonely part of me, love her, accept her and know that it's okay and normal to be lonely—it means I'm not a robot. Far from it, I'm a lover who wants the opportunity to share all the love I have to give. To a man, to my children, to my family, the one I have yet to create. But it's coming, it's my destiny, I know it, and I will do my best to be patient and trust that when the time is right it will be so.

MARCH 17

Quite the day. I got a new idea for my radio show while I was in the shower, so I took it in almost a completely different direction than what I had planned last night. The new version felt more authentic and had a better flow. I started out talking about my ongoing exploration into what gets in the way of the flow of love and about the focus of this week, which was on money. I talked about sacred economics and even played the audio of the film. I talked about bridging the two worlds of money and gifting and said that from the fusion of the two, something even better would emerge. I shared my vision for the world and invited others to do the same, then I brought in some magic from a song I played.

As I'm writing this, I'm feeling kind of detached from it, like my heart isn't in it. Like I'm reporting on my day again.

What's really going on for me right now is that I'm facing the reality of my loneliness. I just got a tarot reading from a new friend and potential roommate regarding questions around relationship, "What's in the way?" and "How do I shift the disconnect that I feel around relationship?"

We did a specific spread for relationship. We focussed on a guy who I've been seeing and have felt a little frustrated about. Feeling like he hasn't been as available and as present as I would like. But interestingly enough, the cards showed that even though his energy is going out in many directions, he is ready for love. The first row is about him, the second row about me and the third about us together. Three cards came up for him (you keep pulling cards until you get a Major Arcana), the first card was the 'Five of Discs,' the second, 'The Lovers' and the third, 'Queen of Cups.' I only had one card, and it was the 'Prince of Wands,' a lot of fire, activity, ferocity—from the image, I felt as if no one would want to approach me because it looks quite dangerous, fire spikes flying out in all directions. Fascinating. The cards for both of us were 'Ace of Wands,' which was quite magical and evoked a sense of connection, passion, synergy, union. The next card was 'Five of Cups,' or disappointment, which is how I often feel in the areas of relationship, sex and money. The final card was 'The Star,' which evoked the sense of magic, flow, destiny, peace, trust.

I mentioned that I saw aloneness in the card, which got us on that topic, and it came out how my deepest fear is of being alone. I asked what to do about that, how to get beyond that, so she had me pull another card, and I pulled the 'Ten of Cups.' That evoked a sense of receptivity, abundance, flow, light and connection. We talked about how perhaps what I need to do is allow the loneliness to be a part of me and, that in the acceptance of it, I become whole rather than needing to get rid of the loneliness. The loneliness is a part of me, and I haven't been willing to fully accept it and have felt a lot of shame about it. I notice that I haven't revealed that part of myself to James (the man I've been seeing, and I'm giving him that name to make it easier to talk about him). Last night we talked and, when he asked how I was, I said, "Good" and "Life was full," and I shared nothing about the loneliness I had been feeling, for fear of scaring him away. Not wanting to come across as needy. But I see there's a risk of becoming, or at least coming across as being, too fiercely independent.

Today's theme or life lesson is to be more present and to have more acceptance of what is. It came from all angles: Destiny Tarot from my friend, Claudia; Enneagram; Stephen Cope's book; my tarot reading. My own intuition. It's my practice for this time in my life: be present, stop fantasizing and getting caught up in my visions for the future, stop trying to make things happen. Be still and receptive. Allow and trust.

MARCH 18

I'm at a loss of what to say. My mind is a jumble of so many things. Sometimes I go through phases where so much happens in such a short time that I can't seem to track it all. It's all a big whirl inside my head, and I can't seem to think straight or make sense of it all. So much seems to have happened. I've already said that. It's almost like a wormhole or like I move into hyperspeed or—what do they say in Star Trek? Oh yeah, warp speed. It's times like these when I start to wonder about my sanity. I feel quite calm and functional on one level, but I feel that if I tried to explain everything that I'm experiencing, I'd be thought to be crazy. I'm trying to make sense of it all and I just can't. It's like my brain doesn't have the neuroreceptors, or what have you, to process everything. Now I feel like I'm being dramatic, when really it's not all that big of a deal. I've just been going through some deep internal churning of stuff: past, present and future. Getting to see how much I don't actually live in the present and how much I live in my head, fretting about the past or fantasizing about the future.

This morning in Kirtan I felt or recognized that mechanism in me that keeps me separate and feeling alone. At the same time, I was having these weird thoughts that we are all truly alone if we all come from the 'One Source' and then, through our singing, I was feeling the connection to all of the people in the space. I'm having emotion come up out of frustration of not feeling able to express or capture my experience in words. Now my breath has sped up, and it sounds like I'm almost panting. I'm feeling uncomfortable being in my body, like I'm touching on something forbidden or ... I can't find the words, so much emotion and thoughts flowing through me and sensation. I feel confused and sad and uncertain and lost and in pain, and I don't know what to do about it all. It brings up that familiar fear that "I'll be alone for the rest of my life" because no one would want to be with someone so 'fucked up.' I'm scared and wondering if anyone will ever read this and, if so, will you care or think I'm really strange, pathetic even. Or is this happening for a reason, so that I write these words to serve a purpose to help you in some way, to make a difference? Or is it all pointless and meaningless like I read about in Stephen Cope's book, that yoga truly begins at the point of despair when there is no hope and everything seems meaningless? I don't understand. What's it all for? My life, what's it for? Is any purpose that I come up with or imagine, just that, a fabric of my imagination, just to feel or seem important. Am I supposed to care or not care? Reveal my loneliness or try to be strong? Am I the only one plagued by these questions? Does anyone else have any inkling of what I'm going through? They must. In fact, it would be arrogant to think otherwise.

Sometimes I feel like such a child, clueless, out of my realm. Like I'm trying to pretend to be this grown up that knows what she's doing and, really, I don't have a clue and I'm not even very good at the pretending. In fact, I suck. And I feel like people look at me and think "Is she ever going to grow up?" and "What's her problem?" I think about my parents and all the responsibility that they have, and it just boggles my mind. Am I just simple? And yet I feel so complex. It could be that I just have a different path.

My friend, Claudia, said, that according to my 'destiny birth card,' I constantly struggle so that I keep being guided or driven to deeper spirituality. That resonated with me because it seems like I can't get things figured out, such as the career, money, material realm stuff. I do to a certain degree, but I can't seem to get beyond a certain point. Yeah, it's like I keep being called upon to dig deeper into faith and trust, and my connection to Spirit/God/the Mystery—what have you.

I still don't know what to call it/s/he. Mostly I use the Mystery, in my thinking or prayers. Sometimes I use 'the Divine.' Sometimes Spirit or God. Sometimes Source. And yet I feel that connection eludes me, too. I've had fleeting moments of grace in which I have felt deeply connected but not enough to be unshakeable in my faith. I want to help, I want to be of service, I want to fulfill my life's purpose. I just don't know exactly what it is yet, if there even is such a thing.

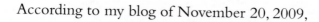

According to my blog of November 20, 2009,

> I know my mission, I know who I am, I am love unbound, here to inspire, touch, ignite, awaken and open others to their truest essence and potential. I am here to join together with others to celebrate life and live it to the fullest! I will stop at nothing, nothing can deter me, stop me, distract me or interfere with me. It is impossible, for it is my destiny.

How could I be so sure then and so 'not sure' now? Fascinating, I shake my head and wonder who that person was, and where did she go? Was that just my ego? A naïve hopeful part of me that needed to die? Or is she still in me somewhere, just waiting to reemerge?

As I paused for a bit from writing and let my mind wander, a thought came to me, "When life gets too full and complicated, I start to go crazy, that's why I have been doing so well on Cortes, the simple life." My nervous system calms down, and my mind is less stimulated. I can just take it day by day, and when I thought about my coming week and how busy and full it seems, I started to feel anxious and thought I just want to be a stay-at-home mom. I know that's probably just a fantasy and that being a mom is super-crazy busy and full and, at times, that's why I question whether I could truly be a mom. I'm in overthinking mode. I need to just stop, go and meditate and get some sleep. It's getting late anyway. Thanks for listening. If anything, I hope this helped you feel a little less crazy than you maybe thought you were. *That you're not alone in your perceived craziness! ;-)*. Or at the very least provided some amusement. I need to remember that more, the humour piece! It's so integral to remember to laugh at myself. But crying is good too and, in case you didn't know, I just did a lot of that while I was writing. It actually felt good to get it out. "Better out than in," they say! ;-) Until next time. Goodnight.

MARCH 19

Amazing how quickly life can change, kind of like the weather of late. Ever feel like the weather is reflecting your inner world or vice versa? The nurse I saw today even said that she felt people were being affected by the weather; a lot of people have been feeling unsettled and a sense of restlessness. This morning I awoke to a snow blizzard which shifted to blue sky and sunshine within an hour then back to flurries and back to sunshine and then shifted to heavy gusts of wind and rain. My head is spinning just talking about it. Wow, the wind is really picking up now. The whole house is shaking. May have another power outage. It's amazing how the weather can totally throw a wrench in plans and can really let me know how fragile and susceptible we are to the forces of nature.

I had a good day of sharing my gifts and connecting authentically. It felt sweet and fulfilling to be sharing my bodywork with people in the community who really benefited from it. If I hadn't offered a trade, I might not have had the chance to share and connect with them in that way. I feel like I haven't had any new awareness around money to share, except I do remember now that during my Quantum Light Breath Meditation, I had a thought about offering a 'life coaching' program called Thrive Alive and was trying to work out how to offer it. Should I do it for free for a limited time or to limited people or charge a fee with the option for people to pay? Or I guess if I were to do it by my declaration, I would offer it to whoever wanted to join in and would leave it open as to what and how they gave back in return. That would be my act of faith. I'm still trying to manage my finances and work it all out to make it 'fair' and to feel like I'm being 'valued.'

QUANTUM LIGHT BREATH

Developed by Jeru Kabbal in the early nineties, the *Quantum Light Breath* is a breathing meditation process that accelerates personal transformation by releasing withheld feelings and revealing unconscious programs. It is designed to take participants into an expanded state of consciousness and ultimately into blissful embodiment. Here, Universal Love is experienced as a natural reality, not as an unreachable concept, where there is a deep connection to the Universal Intelligence. *Quantum Light Breath* participants often describe "Satori," or awakening experiences during the practice.[15]

The Quantum Light Breath is the most efficient process
I have encountered to cleanse the soul and inspire
creativity.
I highly recommend it as a daily meditation.
~ Margot Anand

If I just knew that what I have to offer is valuable, and I offered it trusting that I would receive exactly what I needed in return, in theory and in faith, it would all work out. That would be in integrity. It scares me to do it that way. Thoughts abound such as, "I'll screw up my reputation, devalue myself" and "I won't make any money" and "I won't make a living" and "People won't take me seriously." But I'm really getting that it all doesn't matter. I do offer value; I have a lot to offer that will greatly serve and benefit others, and I have this intuition, this knowing that I will be taken care of. It's almost like the law of physics. Maybe I'm being naïve or idealistic, but I'll never find out unless I try it. I could be bitter and jaded and not even try but where's the fun in that?!

One of the biggest blocks for me, to really offering all that I have to give, is the logistics of charging money. I find it all so complicated, a game that's not any fun. So I'm creating a new game—well, maybe it's not new but new for me. I have the impulse to offer myself in service to others, so why not just offer and trust and allow flow to happen? Part of me thinks this is a copout; maybe it is. But I don't think so. Yes, I am avoiding the whole selling myself thing, but that's the whole point. Selling is not what I want my life to be about. I don't want to sell myself. I want to offer and share and give and contribute and trust and allow and receive and offer and share and give some more and allow the natural flow to happen. It's all about intention, right? There's no right or wrong way to do anything. There is living life by my heart's calling and being in integrity with my values and with the things that are important to me. That's how I want to live my life. That's how I am choosing to live my life. It's scary but good. So be it!

Anyone want to sign up for my Thrive Alive program? ;-) I'll do everything in my power to help and support you to live your life in accordance with your values, to follow your heart and to live your truth. I have no idea what that will look like, but together we will explore the possibilities and see what wants to unfold. I don't have the answers. I help you find them out for yourself. I offer you my love, respect, energy, support, presence, care and curiosity. I ask for your willingness, openness, trust and commitment. I was going to add, "And whatever you feel it is worth to you," BUT that would be asking for something in return. AND to be totally honest and transparent, I do have hopes that you will express your gratitude with something in return AND I am trusting that it will all work out. Isn't life wild, fun and hilarious?! The great mystery … gotta love it! Blessings on your journey wherever it takes you.

MARCH 20

Amazing things are happening. I've been having mass epiphanies. Spring is springing! I'm at my friend and dear soul sistar's for an equinox gathering. I've spent an evening of connecting, sharing, feasting, dancing, expanding, loving, expressing. It's one of those mass opening and expansive events. I smoked some hash that was locally made in the snow this past winter. The offer felt too special an opportunity to pass up even though I had quit smoking any mind-altering substances back in September. When it was offered, I got a big yes so I went with it. I don't like living with rigidity or strict rules. I like making decisions in the moment based on my heart and body and soul. When faced with decisions, I like to base my choice on: "What will bring more aliveness?" *This is a teaching I received from Satyen at the workshop, Money Mastery.*

I was and am still hesitant to share about smoking the hash with you, a small fear of being judged or made wrong. But my commitment is to be transparent and honest, as fully as possible. I've been seeing tonight that this can be challenging for me and that I have been holding back, hiding. Perhaps out of shyness or insecurity. I suspect the fear of rejection has an influence on how much I don't share. When something is offered from a magical being dressed in white lace, petticoat and a giant flower hat, I accept. *Wouldn't you? ;-)* We went outside, the stars were just starting to shine. One star was a massive shining ball of light. My friend said it must be a planet, possibly Pluto. She then offered me a beautifully glass-blown dragon pipe of the magical concoction. I set my intention for my heart, body and mind to open and inhaled.

Shortly after my mind began to expand, my heart opened and my body relaxed. My breath deepened, I felt myself become more present as if fully occupying the space that is my body and seeing more clearly through my eyes and feeling more fully with my heart. I began to see and feel how amazing my life is, how blessed I am to live in this incredible place with these phenomenal people. I came to see that I haven't been fully allowing or embracing all the wonder and beauty I am surrounded by. I also came to see how much I have been holding inside. I ended up gushing praise and love to my friends who were with me, fully taking the opportunity to acknowledge them for how lovely they are, how much I have appreciated them being in my life and for how welcome they made me feel when I arrived on the island. They made me feel like I belonged by being helpful and encouraging. I felt really good fully expressing my appreciation and praise, and it was true and real and lovely. Fulfillment.

I came in and danced and felt myself alive and glowing with love and joy. At one point I was drawn to the fire next to my friend's 3-year-old daughter. She was lying on the futon looking incredibly adorable. I couldn't help but shower her with affection. I rubbed her back and her legs, caressed her face and ended up kissing her all over. I would ask where else she wanted a kiss, and she would point to her cheek or her chin or raise her hand. It was the most precious and delightful time, my heart was exploding with enamouredness. It was definitely 'delightenment' at its finest.

A master in the art of living draws no sharp distinction between his work
and his play; his labor and his leisure; his mind and his body; his education
and his recreation. He hardly knows which is which. He simply pursues his
vision of excellence through whatever he is doing, and leaves others
to determine whether he is working or playing. To himself, he always appears to be doing both.
~ Francois Auguste Rene Chateaubriand

I have so much I want to share with you now. So much that it's hard to capture. Where to go next? A deep breath, a sigh, a softening of my jaw and face, neck and shoulders. I allow my mind to open. I was sharing with my pixie friend about the journey I'm on with exploring sacred economics: what that means to me and what I've been discovering. I shared with her one of the epiphanies I had while sitting in front of the fire. I realized that this experiment, this journey, is helping me open up and share more, share more freely and generously and spontaneously and that the money transaction 'thang' gets in the way of me sharing. I get too in my head about things, and I end up not offering what I genuinely want to offer from my heart because I don't know how to go about arranging the transaction. All the concern and worry that come with that—anxiousness even—they block my flow. I truly see and believe that this way of offering—genuinely, spontaneously, fully, freely, openly, generously—is the way of being for me. I'm living fully in faith and trust that I will be taken care of and always have what I need.

I am feeling very excited about life, and it's not just the hash. ;-) I am surrounded by incredible beings with shared vision and values, and we believe in magic and possibility, and we are creating our lives together, in love and joy and gratitude. This is the life that I have dreamed of, and I am living it more and more every day—the more I open up and allow it to happen. My friends were saying that this is the golden age, and we are creating it.

Part of me is starting to wonder how much I am going into fantasy. Is anything truly possible? At times it feels like it is; at other times I'm not so sure. Nearby my dear soul brother, J, is rap battling with the kids; it's really awesome. He says it's called a cypher. We're all just chillin', some of the kids are playing games on the computer, some of the ladies are doing tarot on the rug, a sweet young lass is sitting next to me being my muse with her precious innocence. She's asking me what I'm doing, and I told her; she says that it's really cool and that I type really fast. I'm getting a little tired now and feeling like it's time to rejoin the party, so I'm going to bid adieu. Exciting times, still lots to tell. Will get to it again soon.

I'm home now, after a spot of nettle tea and a card from the Inner Child Tarot. I pulled the 'Pied Piper, Guide of Wands.' All about imagination, the muse of creativity and inspiration, childlike innocence, the inner guide/knowing. It said to sing, dance and play. So

Shaeah Love : **101**

bang on. It even talked about the townspeople not valuing the Pied Piper and his services and not being willing to pay him until they come around to see his gift and contribution. Then they were able to appreciate and value him. I believe this is symbolic of the journey I'm on. At first I might be met with resistance, disbelief or judgment, but I know that people will come to see my pure intention and heart, will naturally open to receive and appreciate what I have to offer and will give back in some way or pay it forward. I trust the flow of the Universe.

Earlier this evening, my pixie sistar had been sharing a realization she had had during her travels, that we are only limited by our imagination. I get this notion at times, too. One of my teachers, Satyen, once said, "If you can think it, it is possible." At one point today, I could see how my life reflects the amount I am willing to expand and include. All of life and its aspects are available to be experienced. It's up to me what I choose to receive or experience and, yet as I write this, I realize that's not completely true because there is the mystery factor: life will throw curve balls. Well, hmmm, that's not contradictory. It just implies that yes, life will bring us things we don't want or expect. We can try to resist those things and try to deny them, but I'm pretty sure that's what creates suffering. One of the ways suffering is created anyway. My understanding is that trying to resist and also trying to force anything or anyone are the two most significant, or should I say, 'common' ways to cause suffering. I guess that's where cause and effect come into play.

I'm simultaneously aware of the reasons I enjoyed partaking in plant medicines and also why I didn't enjoy it. My mind expands, and I feel like I tap into some greater consciousness and download all of these amazing realizations. But the problem is that my mind eventually contracts again, and I begin to question whether what I opened up to was true or fantasy. I start to doubt and wonder what is truly real. Like now, a voice is coming in and asking, "What about surrender," and I'm laughing because that's exactly what I'm talking about, but from a different angle.

I see now that it's all the same thing. Acceptance of life. Gratitude for what is. The expansion is the capacity to hold it all. It's all there, so it's up to me how much I allow myself to open and surrender to what is. My refusal or inability to open and allow is what causes me to suffer. I could feel myself more open even in my yoga practice today, so it wasn't just the hash. It's a culmination of a lot of things. Being honest and vulnerable with the man I am dating was a big part of it. The sessions I gave yesterday got my energy flowing. Spending quality time with good-hearted loving people and taking time to just be with myself in a space of acceptance and curiosity are also a part of it. I feel all that I have learned over my lifetime(s) is finally being integrated and lived.

Whoa, I just looked at the time, it's after 1am. The latest I've been up in a while but, as the 'Guide of Wands' said, "One never knows when the muse will come and when the muse will be gone, so carpe diem!" As long as it's flowing, keep going! ;-) Hee hee, like my rhyme? I didn't even try. This is the kind of writing I like, it flows and is fun and playful. I feel like my writing over the past while has been a bit heavy and that's okay because that's what was real and true, but I do see myself feeling better about sharing my happy times. I have been quite sad, and another realization I had tonight is, yeah, I get sad when I'm alone sometimes and that's perfectly natural. I like connecting and sharing with people and, when I'm not, I feel lonely sometimes. It doesn't make the amazingness of my life any less. It's just part of my experience of life, and that's the key—just part of it, not all of it. My sadness doesn't discount the good. Remember, it's all about expansion, holding it all, not either or. That's SARK's message, the 'marvelous messy middle,' the place that includes it all and gives a person space to feel more than one thing and the different feelings may even seem contradictory, but it just is.

Like today, I was disappointed that Ashley (*the woman that was considering being my roommate*) decided not to move to Cortes, and I was also genuinely wanting to be supportive of her choice and her life's path so I wished her well. I really do love my life. I feel so blessed and at times am in awe of all the incredible blessings I am surrounded by and filled with. This island is magic, or perhaps it's life that is magic, and I'm just able to tap into it more here. Or perhaps it's me who is magic, and my life and this island are the outer reflection of that. How's that for a mind, frick?! I suspect it's a combo of all of the above. Yes, yes and yes. I loved the yes game in theatre, actually it was 'yes let's.' Okay, I think I need to sleep now, a big yawn, and my eyes are getting droopy. Sweetest of dreams.

I'll share with you what I say to myself before I go to sleep. My mom taught it to me, "I will have a peaceful and restful sleep with pleasant and joyful dreams that will completely ___." You fill the blank. I usually say, "... that will completely rejuvenate, renew and refresh my whole being." If you have a cold or feel unwell, you can say, "That will completely restore my health." So be it. Bonne nuit.

From My
Heart
To Yours

MARCH 21

I just got my ass kicked by a movie called *Soul Surfer*, or should I say 'soul kicked.' ;-) It definitely took me by surprise. I wasn't expecting much from it except some nice Hollywood fluff. It's profoundly moving and inspiring. It was a lot about faith and strength of spirit. I feel myself being drawn closer to God, and this scares me. A deeper and deeper faith is being called upon from within me. I marvel at what people are capable of, such strength of spirit. Certainly puts things in perspective. The movie had some amazing one liners in it; I'm almost tempted to watch it again just to capture them. The support she received from her family and community to find her way was brilliant. If everyone received that level of love, support and encouragement, we would live in a completely different world.

MARCH 25

I guess I took a bit of a hiatus from writing. Not intentionally. Life just happened. Which is a good thing. I've been really engaged in life, connecting a lot with friends, being involved and participating in my community. It's been amazing actually. Full, rich, sweet, fun, enlivening … I guess that's the energy of spring: new life, fresh shoots, budding flowers of friendship and connection. Very sweet indeed. I just returned from a glorious walk through the woods after lying on the beach soaking up the warmth and energy of the sun and having some great conversations with my dear friend, Andrea, who is visiting from the big city. She loves it here. In fact, she talked about living here even before she arrived. I knew she would. She's another soul sister who shares the same values and passions.

I'm really enjoying connecting and sharing with people lately. I feel more at ease within myself and able to share more openly and freely. It feels good. I feel good. I wonder how much is connected to my journey with sacred economics, how much is the natural evolution of my being and how much is simply due to it being spring. Probably a combination of all of the above.

I'm having concern come up about me and this book. I guess we are one in the same; the book is a reflection of where I am at in life. Insecurities are coming up, doubt, uncertainty. Having thoughts that I'm being naïve and foolish by thinking this will fly. Feeling nervous about exposing myself so fully. Concerned about being judged and thought poorly of. Why does it matter so much? Why do I feel that I need to prove myself? Feel that I need recognition or approval from an outside source? I wish I could be confident and sure of myself, 'self-assured,' I guess you might call it.

Sometimes I feel like I have the maturity level of a 12-year old, not to diss 12-year olds. I think they're great, that's probably why I like to act like them. ;-) But I seriously do feel at times like I have a developmental problem or issue. Now, I'm feeling ridiculous, as if I'm looking for pity or something, but I'm not. At least I don't think I am. Maybe I am. Who knows what I do unconsciously? That's why it's unconscious. Instead of impressing you, I'm … what? What am I doing? Being honest. I guess that's the whole point of this book, of my life, to be real and honest as much as I can. To stop hiding, stop pretending. I'm not perfect. I don't have it all together. I screw up. I make mistakes. I say stupid stuff. I do silly things. I regret. I hurt. I get scared, a lot, and cry, and I also laugh a lot, especially at myself, at how ridiculous I can be. I marvel at life and others. I take joy in the beauty of nature and people. I love children and how sweet they can be, and I am appalled at how nasty they are at times. How sweet and nasty we can all be. I don't understand life at all, but I find enjoyment of it more and more. Sometimes I love life and sometimes I hate it, and the same goes for myself. Sometimes I love myself and see myself as beautiful and amazing and, other times, I see myself through cruel, critical and judging eyes and think I'm one of the world's greatest losers. Fascinating! Truly, it boggles my mind, or perhaps it's my mind that boggles me! Hee hee, that's pretty clever. ;-)

I really enjoy those times when I amuse myself. That's the best. When I make myself smile, like right now, and I get that feeling like it's all okay. None of it really matters that much. I'm here, I'm alive, I haven't killed anyone. I do my best to be a good person and to make the world a better place even if it's in small ways. Sure I've got big ideas, big visions, but it's what I do on a day-to-day basis that matters, right? How I treat the people I meet, the choices I make. It's funny, I'm looking at a picture of me on my laptop smiling a big goofy smile, and I see someone who is happy and sweet and pretty, even with my wrinkles and off-white teeth and a scar. With all my imperfections, I'm pretty okay. I'm a good egg, as my uncle would say. I wonder if that will ever completely sink in? Will I ever get past self-consciousness, insecurity and self-loathing? Somehow I suspect it will always be there to some degree but will fade like a scar fades over time.

I was talking to my friend about this anomaly during our walk today, asking her why she thinks a lot—perhaps all—of us struggle with the issue of self-love and acceptance. She figures it's what keeps us motivated to grow and improve ourselves. But I wonder if that would be possible to do and perhaps would be even way more enjoyable from a place of pure curiosity and enthusiasm rather than from the need to 'fix' or 'change' ourselves.

I once got, in a Clearing session, that one of my fixed attitudes is 'there's something wrong,' and that attitude creates a filter through which I see myself and everything around me. I had this major shift and moment of liberation when I came to see that the things I thought were wrong, were actually not a problem and could instead become a project. This allowed for excitement, curiosity and enthusiasm for those areas rather than the heaviness and shame that I had been feeling instead. Sometimes I forget about that little revelation and start to see things as a problem again, but when I catch myself and shift to seeing my life as a project again, I relax and am able to enjoy myself.

I'm feeling the need or desire to talk about a woman who has helped me a lot in my life. She was the one who did that Clearing session for me where I realized that life's problems weren't problems anymore but projects. This session was during the last time I almost gave up my will to live, last spring. The reason I'm feeling the need to talk about her is because she is someone who believed in me. She truly saw something good in me and wanted to—and actually did—help me to see that for myself. She has a huge heart of compassion, and I feel so much love and gratitude to her for all her years of support and real help. God bless you, Anjali! You are a compassionate, generous, caring, loving soul, and I love and appreciate you with my whole heart and being. I dedicated 8 years of my life in service to her, not solely, but as much as I could. I am honoured and humbled to know someone who is so real and who gives so much. She did, and does, great work and has helped and served hundreds, maybe thousands, of people.

I've been lucky to have had some really great teachers and mentors. At times, I remember thinking or wishing I had teachers who were more renowned or famous, but I love that they were real people just doing their best to make a difference in people's lives. Their work was about love and truth and about being of service. These people changed my life. In fact, at times, I feel like I owe them my life. Again, they saw something in me and believed in me when I didn't and, through their ongoing love, support, encouragement, mentorship, friendship and contact, I gradually came to believe in myself and see what they saw, mostly. At times, I still don't understand what they saw or why they took me under their wing and, at other times, I think how lucky they were to have me! ;-) I guess and hope that we mutually benefitted. We became quite the force actually. A motley crew of spiritual warriors. I love that we were so humanly imperfect and tried our damnedest to wake up as many people as possible. We all shared the same passion of liberation. I remember when I fell in love with Anjali and Satyen (*the founder of the spiritual growth company I worked for*). It was at my first Enlightenment/Illumination Intensive where I had my first taste of liberation. They seemed like true wizards sitting at the front of the room, seemingly larger than life and glowing with passion and rawness. I swore that I would go wherever they went. And I did for the next 8 years of my life, with a few pit stops on the way. I tasted freedom, and I knew instantly that I wanted to help others experience it, too. So I did.

For to be free is not merely to cast off one's chains, but to live in a way that respects and enhances the freedom of others.
~ Nelson Mandela

Hmmm, I guess I do have some power. I do follow through with choices, can make commitments and have loyalty, dedication and perseverance. Most of the time, I don't see those things in myself. Most of the time, I see someone who has mostly failed and has nothing to show for her life. Fascinating. You may have noticed that's one of my favourite words—fascinating. It's just that I marvel at life a lot; it truly does perplex me often.

Anyway, I'm starting to fade. I've shared a lot and, yes, still have so much more. Patience, dear Padawan. That's another one of my biggest practices right now, I'm pretty sure I've mentioned that. Patience. I put on my cloak of patience and lie me down to sleep. Good night.

MARCH 28

This being human is a guest house. Every morning is a new arrival. A joy, a depression, a meanness, some momentary awareness comes as an unexpected visitor ... Welcome and entertain them all. Treat each guest honorably. The dark thought, the shame, the malice, meet them at the door laughing, and invite them in. Be grateful for whoever comes, because each has been sent as a guide from beyond.

~ Rumi

Warning, the following is not pretty: raw, real, ugly stuff. Stuff is being stirred up, and the shit is starting to hit the fan. Prepare to get messy. I'm really going through it right now. This is one of those moments that I predicted, where I don't want you to know or see. I want to hide this part of me. I feel ashamed. It's linked to my sacred economics journey.

I hit a wall around attachment and expectations today. I'm having trouble writing about this and am wanting to just make excuses, to not talk about it and to just hide. I feel ashamed and embarrassed. I don't like admitting that my faith is faltering and that I can't just give without expectation. I feel like I'm failing and that I can't do this. I find myself making excuses such as, "People aren't ready for this" and "People don't value something if they don't pay" and "I'm not valued if I don't charge money." I have feelings of being taken advantage of, resentment, fear. I feel contracted, like I'm closing off. I'm questioning whether I do have value. I felt a lot of sadness and anger processing with my friend earlier today about this. She totally called me on my shit and said that I'm not living up to my commitment and my word of no expectation and that I'm being totally attached—and she's right. Argh!

I have a lot of sadness and anger up right now. I'm seeing and experiencing limiting beliefs. I expressed to my friend, "That people aren't ready for this."

When she asked me, "What people?"

I kept saying, "People."

She kept pushing and asking, "What people?"

When I finally said, "Me," a rush of anger came up, and I had to scream.

I feel upset and frustrated and disappointed. I feel like I can't do this. Thoughts come up that if people don't pay, they don't get value, they won't receive value, they'll even block it. If I don't get paid, I don't feel valued. I feel taken advantage of and used and underappreciated. I feel a lot of sadness when I write that. This is super uncomfortable and feels super icky. Bleh. I am hating myself right now, and I don't know why. I feel like I'm a nobody, that I don't matter, that I can't make a difference, that nobody cares about me, fuckinglkajf;oi ej;oaine;voina;obin;oinealke v;inaeoinbean.ldknbo;aeiv dwieg[3209gn'vjv'eponblewm90j2 gpeobjriaejfgjq3049ngoinrg;oi. Arghhhhhhhhhhh!!!!!! So much anger!!!!! I just want to swear and kick and scream. My body hurts. My jaw aches. I feel pressure in my head. Tears are streaming down my face, and I'm thinking there's no fucking way anyone is going to see this and, if they did, they'd laugh and think I was an idiot anyway. This whole book, my whole life is a waste of time and energy. Big sobs now. I want to be brilliant and loved and liked and admired by all, and it feels impossible and stupid. And pointless.

I feel a sense of relief, a big release. Space has opened in my chest. I need to blow my nose. Snot was dripping. Now I'm chuckling at myself. I'm not sure I know how to fully trust, and this saddens me. My right shoulder really hurts and that's usually an indication that I'm 'efforting' too much, using too much will. Or it could just simply be that I've over exerted it in yoga and by giving massage. Perhaps a combo.

I notice it's difficult to receive. I feel guilty about the money my friend gave me for food and a massage and then, on the other hand, I feel resentful about someone else not giving me enough money. I feel caught between a rock and a hard place. Guilt and resentment.

Two very ugly places. Damned if I do, damned if I don't. I feel guilty sometimes when I do receive money and resentful sometimes when it doesn't feel like enough. Part of me wants to have the freedom and choices that a lot of money brings; another part doesn't want to care and would rather just have a simple, happy life. I don't think money is wrong or bad; it's just the energy and meaning that we attach to it that distorts it. And I obviously have attached a lot of meaning to money and to what it represents and signifies.

When my friend was coaching me through the trigger and upset, she asked me to recall my intention for this journey, which was "to live with integrity with my heart's calling to give my gifts generously. As an act of faith and to flush out limiting beliefs that I have around sharing my gifts." She pointed out that I was succeeding in this latter intention. This is the icky part. I feel great and wonderful when I'm just giving, sharing and living with faith and trust, which is how it's been the last week or so. But as soon as I hit up against one of those beliefs ... yuck! I have to remember it's a part of the journey, an opportunity for new awareness, consciousness, an opportunity to make new choices. Purifying, clearing, creating space for new possibilities. Knowing that, it still doesn't seem to make it easier for me. But I do know I'll get through this, and something surprising may be on the other side. I'll let you know if and when I get there.

It's all just coming up today. For the last week or so, I've just been really engaged in life and enjoying myself with little or no thought of money. It's almost the midway point of this experiment, and I haven't had much money flow in, but I have had an abundance of other things, especially connections.

I'm still having trouble expressing this, and I'm not sure why. It makes me think I'm avoiding or trying to hide something. Trying to sound good or impress you. I just want to be honest. "What's really going on?" I ask myself. The essence is that I'm struggling with trust and faith. Why can't I just give freely and trust like I hope to?

The guy I was seeing dumped me last night, too, to add salt to injury. Although I felt relieved because I knew deep down he couldn't be present and wasn't available for a relationship. He didn't dump me because I suck; he just doesn't have energy or time for a relationship right now. He's going through a really difficult time and says he needs time to get strong and heal. It's starting to really storm outside again. We may lose power again. Anyway, part of me trusts that if we are meant to be, it'll happen when it's time. Or space is being created for someone else better suited to come in to my life. Of course, I'm disappointed but not as much as I thought I'd be. Maybe I trust more than I think. I don't know. Money and men!! Why so much struggle with both?! So frustrating.

I'm just realizing I totally changed subjects. Not sure if I'm avoiding the money topic or if it's just that they are so linked. Let's look and see and make sure I've explored and expressed everything about this issue. I close my eyes, take a few deep breaths, feel, open, allow, listen and see what comes up. What's there is that I'm tired and feel sadness. A feeling like I just want to give up. I want to be held and consoled and told that everything's going to be all right. I want to be saved. I give a cynical chuckle under my breath and shake my head, "Not this fucking thing again." It's embarrassing. I feel ashamed again. I can't do it on my own. I can't and don't know how to do this thing called life on my own. I can't figure it out. I don't know what to do and how to do it. I need help and I don't know how to get it, who to ask, how, where, when? I still feel like I'm trying to prove something, earn something, get something, and I imagine voices shouting back, "Of course, that's what life is about." I feel subtle disgust. Tightness in my chest, jaw and belly. Why can't I just be normal? Like other people, get a job and live a simple life. Why do I have to make it so difficult and complicated for myself? I would so love and welcome ignorant bliss right now.

My friend and I were talking about suffering last night, how it's so prevalent and it seems there's no escaping it. If we have material wealth, we most often still suffer through our minds with habitual thoughts of 'something's missing' or from guilt or shame, and there's the suffering of starvation or war on such a large scale that so many people are affected by. I can't see how I could ever get to a place where I'm not feeling or aware of suffering because, if my life is going great, others are still suffering and, if we are connected, how could I not feel their suffering. If I improve my life and lessen my suffering, though, at least there's less suffering in the world.

Why do I have this fucking crazy overthinking, analyzing mind? It won't stop! I've been super active and involved in life and community, and that doesn't prevent my mind from going to crazy places in the times of stillness and silence. I can't stay active 24/7. "It's what I choose to focus on," my mind says as I watch a deer strut across my lawn. Practice presence, gratitude, breath, awareness, openness. All the things that I teach, of course! "We teach what we most need to learn." Fascinating. Frustrating!

I'm hungry, need to go eat. I feel a little Neanderthal-ish now. Aren't I pretty?! One of my friends told me the other day, when I asked her what true love was, that it's letting go of all expectations and loving and accepting someone just as they are, shadow and dark side included. I guess this is my opportunity to expose and love those sides of myself.

My friend, Andrea, made an interesting observation of me. She thinks that I'm more naturally an introvert, that I just think I'm an extrovert or think I should be and that actually being with people too often drains me. I've had this thought myself. Wondered which I truly am. I definitely need my solo time to recharge and replenish. She said this is the determining factor, where we get our energy from. But then, I think about times when I'm dancing and feeling tired, and all I have to do is shift my focus to someone else and, from that connection, I get energy and inspiration. So I'm not so sure. It's all labels and boxes anyway.

I did grow up mostly on my own and spent a lot of time by myself or with my pets. I remember long walks in the woods, I think I've mentioned this before. Did I mention that my memory is a bit off? ;-) So you may hear a few things more than once. I guess that'll get ironed out in the editing or maybe not—depends how raw and real I leave it. That's one of the main intentions and purposes of this book, to be as transparent as possible, so we'll see how it all pans out.

I'm wiped. I was supposed to go to a Salsa class tonight, but I think I'm staying home and watching movies. I wish I had a tub of ice cream to go with it. I have this deep yearning to be held right now. I wonder how many people live with that feeling and never get it fulfilled. How many longings, wants, desires, and needs don't get fulfilled? Probably way more than I care to imagine. Why does life seem so cruel sometimes? Perplexes me.

APRIL 4

It's been a while. I got off track, distracted. It's my pattern. I start out strong and eventually peter off. I'm not going to let that happen with this book. I'm going to break that pattern, stick to my commitment and see this project through to the end and, even if only one person ever reads it, it will be completed. I'm not sure where to start, so much has been happening. That's one reason I haven't been writing, which in a way is a good thing. I've been really engaged in life. I just turned forty-one yesterday. I had a lovely, magical day. I started out the day with the intention to love myself and let my actions and choices come from that intention. I stayed in bed quite a while, resting and cuddling with my stuffed lion—yes, I'm forty-one and I sleep with a stuffy! ;-) I was laughing at it myself the other night. He's super soft and comforting, and he makes sleeping alone a little less sufferable. Anyway, I asked myself how I wanted my day to start, and the answer was with a bath. So I drew myself a lovely Epsom salt bath with essential oils and candles. Then I nourished myself with yummy food and, by then, the sun had come out. I went for a nice long walk on my favourite circuit. I sat and meditated at the lake for a while. I remember feeling a little sad at that point. I carried on to the waterfall and stood there soaking up those negative ions and letting the rush of flowing water clear away my blues. I splashed some of the crystal clear water on my face, sang the song, "Watching the River Run" *(my mom's favourite Loggins & Messina song)* and reflected on my life. My mood started to lift, then I hugged a giant tree for a while.

Argh, I'm hating my writing, judging it, thinking I'm/it's stupid. I feel tired and cranky. I've had a challenging day emotionally. I felt really sad today when I got up—couldn't stop crying for the longest time and had no idea why. The only thing I could think of was the loneliness factor. Who knows? Does it really matter? I had a great day anyway. Yoga class, a Skype session, taught yoga and gave a bodywork session. Lay in the sun for a while, talked to family, had a bath. There's so much I want to share that's happened, but I'm so tired and unmotivated. I feel that whatever I write will sound lame and be uninspired.

It just feels like time's been moving so fast, so much has been happening and more is just going to keep happening. I don't know how to capture it all or how to choose what to capture. What's important? I think I need to relook at my intentions for this book. Refocus and regroup. I'm starting to feel a little too scattered with it. My main intention is to share openly and honestly from my heart to yours. I'm not sure what the purpose is exactly, but I hope that it will provide a source of inspiration, education, amusement, affirmation. My intention is to speak frankly about the issues and challenges that I am facing in hopes that it will shed some light on what you are experiencing or help you to know that you are not alone or provide insight. I want to provide a living example of true transparency, to give permission to you and others to be free, real and honest.

I feel like I'm talking out of my ass a little, trying to say the right thing. If I'm totally frank, I want to write something so earth-shatteringly profound that people will love it and buy millions of copies so that I can have a nest egg to raise a family. That's it! That's totally the honest truth. It feels really good to say that out loud, to admit that. I'm exploring and demonstrating what it's like to be radically honest. I haven't gotten up the courage to do it in real life yet, face to face with others, so I'm taking the easier way out and starting with the less direct approach in writing with radical honesty first to see how it feels.

It feels really amazing when I nail it on the head, but the funny or odd thing is how difficult that can be. It's wild, it's almost like I'm so conditioned to not speak my absolute bare truth that I don't even know how. Now this is good shit. This is what I'm talking about. Being real, raw, in the moment, baring my soul. Why don't we do this more in life? I've been contemplating that the last few days or so. How much is okay to reveal, to whom, when, and under what circumstances … it's crazy making! Why can't we be just totally and utterly honest in every moment? Why do we have to consider if it's appropriate, what people will think? Who might I offend? What chances will I blow if I speak my truth right now? I have to be careful and watch what I say or do. It's insane! Totally fucked up. I really love and admire people who are bold enough to speak their minds and who do what they feel in the moment. *Have you seen the movie,* The Invention of Lying? *Brilliant film that I highly recommend seeing.* I met a young man like that the other night, I was entranced by him. He had me in stitches, literally on the floor laughing. So refreshing, so free. I asked him how he could be so free at such a young age and he said, "Once you know that you are free and that you can do anything with your mind ... why conform?" Or something like that.

I 'know' that I am free, but some part of me still won't allow myself to be free. And then I get into a mind frick about "am I really free?" How much of my life is predetermined and under some greater force's control and how much free will do I actually have? I really don't know. It's one of my greatest 'issues'—that's not the right word. I think I may have mentioned this already. How much of my life is directed by my own will, how much is by divine will and is there a difference?

It does not do to dwell on dreams, Harry, and forget to live. ~ Professor Dumbledore

Sometimes I get too much in my head about all this, about life. That was the topic of my last radio show, or should I say non-topic. I made it about living life rather than a theme for this exact reason—because sometimes I get too heady about it. That was one of my revelations during an Enlightenment/ Illumination Intensive when I was contemplating 'What is Life?' I got that life is something to be lived not contemplated. I love that. It had me in the aisle laughing my head off, the absurdity of it, the obviousness of it, and how it both invalidated and validated my existence all at the same time. I was obviously given this mind for a reason (ha-ha, no pun intended, but it's actually pretty clever, wouldn't you say?!). And yet, reason seems to interfere with faith or can they be complementary?

Sometimes I feel frustrated by my limited vocabulary. It's from a lack of reading over the last fifteen years of my life. Before that, I was a voracious reader and had an incredibly extensive vocabulary. Oh well, so be it. It's what's so and where I'm at. Have to accept it, just like my fading memory. Things change. I'm glad I got a flow going. I had been feeling so stuck, too caught up in details and wasn't getting to the heart of the matter. The essence, that's what it always comes down to, or it would help if life's circumstances were just about the simple truth. But the opposite is usually true, most often life gets so complicated with details and such that the essence is lost or clouded. But it truly is the essence that is the most ... blah blah blah, I feel like I'm trying to sound all intelligent and wise and shit. Something is there, but I can't capture it at this moment so I gotta just be real about that. I guess that's what I'm trying to do with this book, get to the essence, the heart of the matter, the soul. From my heart to yours, heart to heart, soul to soul. That's what I yearn for. Isn't that what everybody yearns for? That deep connection, pure intimacy.

A question that's been coming up for me about this is, "Is intimacy something that should be saved and only shared with certain people?" Or is my heart and soul best to be shared with all beings, or at least with as many as I can possibly touch? Why hoard or restrict myself? I want to touch as many people as possible and then I ask, "Is that my ego?" I truly feel it's pure generosity of heart and spirit. Yes, of course, some ego part wants recognition, wealth, feelings of importance, validation, and so forth, but the 'essence' is that I want to share my love and my Self generously and openly. That's what feels 'right.' Anything less feels limiting, restrictive or repressive. I'm not talking about having sex with everyone but sharing my essence, my heart, my soul; it wants—I want—to keep expanding and growing to my fullest capacity and then my mind comes in and says, "That's arrogant."

I think I need to stop writing right now. I feel like I'm not making much sense. But I feel that I got some good stuff out, that I finally accessed some real heartfelt sharing. I feel both scared and excited to be sharing like this. I think part of me is still in disbelief or denial that I'll actually share this publicly. Maybe I won't, but a deeper part of me believes I will. I actually initially wrote, "Knows I will," but I changed it to "believes." Hmmm, fascinating I'm still second guessing myself. Oh well, at least I'm being more honest about it and catching myself when I do it.

Thanks for listening. It's funny, but I think it helps to think that someone out there will read this someday. I've heard that it's important to have a witness to your life. In fact, one of my favourite lines from the movie *Shall We Dance* was about that. It was a woman's answer to a question about her husband,

> **We need a witness to our lives. There's a billion people on the planet ... I mean, what does any one life really mean? But in a marriage, you're promising to care about everything ... You're saying 'Your life will not go unnoticed because I will notice it. Your life will not go un-witnessed because I will be your witness.'**

I guess that's why I feel so lonely and sad a lot of the time. I feel like a lot of my life is going by unnoticed or 'unwitnessed.' That's where you come in. So, thanks again. You are playing a very important and powerful role in my life even though you don't know it. I hope you have someone to be a witness to your life. That Ben Harper song just came into my head, "I'm Blessed to Be a Witness" and then I realized that that's most of my life's work, being a witness. Fascinating. Things that make you go hmmm ...

April 8

Easter Sunday. I just got home from an incredible feast with lovely people. I'm experimenting with over-indulging just to have the experience and see what it feels like. It doesn't feel great but, at the same time, it's kind of fun, trying to break out of my body image imprinting. I have a very fixed idea of how my body should look and feel, and I become very self-critical whenever I start to gain any weight or get fleshy in any way. I was thinking tonight as I was going for the second piece of pumpkin pie that it would be healthy for me to embrace being fleshy and claim the ability to feel and be beautiful no matter what my body size. It's been a huge hang up for me. I really admire voluptuous woman who emanate confidence and beauty and who defy the 'beauty myth.' I would love to break free of that imposed idea of how I should look. Speaking of breaking free, that's been a big theme of this week, being Passover and Easter.

My friend Andrea and I have been having a lot of long and in-depth conversations about freedom and life. Today we climbed to Easter Bluff and had a powerful conversation, and we actually did a dyad about value and life choices. I had a profound realization that my life mission is to live from my heart and to allow a pure and authentic expression in each moment. This was very liberating and empowering for me to realize. I don't have to figure out what my mission is as an external expression, that will constantly change and evolve depending on the circumstances and on who I am with. I guess this is the essence I was trying to get at before. It doesn't matter what I do, it's the spirit in which I do it. Is it true? Is it from my heart? Is it in integrity with what my values are and what's important to me? My ideal expression or way of being is that in which I am benefiting both myself and others simultaneously. In fact why live any other way? This is the only way not to perpetuate suffering, either in myself or in others. This is what I aspire to in my life, to live purely and authentically from my heart in a way that is beneficial to myself, others and the earth. In fact, anything less than this is … is what? Unacceptable, but that seems a bit overly dramatic. I'm not sure but it's not 'it.' Perhaps it's an ideal, but really—why live any other way? I know in my heart and my soul that it's possible, and my mission is to prove, or at least to model, that it is possible.

I feel like I'm being arrogant and the thought occurred to me that perhaps that's what everyone else is already doing, and I'm just figuring it out now. I often have this strange feeling that others know something I don't, that they have figured out the great secret to life while I still flounder. But I guess if that were the case, there wouldn't be so much illness created from stress and there wouldn't be so many depressed people.

I had another liberating revelation last week. It's been a powerful time for me. I just have to remember what it was. I pause, close my eyes, take a deep breath. Oh yeah, something in a similar vein, that I don't have to 'figure out' or 'know' who I am or what I am 'supposed to do or be.' In fact, it's better if I don't. That way I give myself permission and freedom to be whatever wants to come through in the moment. Life becomes a journey of discovery, and I get to be surprised by myself all the time. This is when and how real magic happens. This requires a lot of trust and surrender. And, again, that's the way I aspire to live. This gives me the space and freedom to keep expanding into the fullness of my being, to keep exploring the possibilities. I've been trying so hard to figure it/me out. Getting stressed about not knowing and needing to know, putting all this pressure on myself to be something, to do something with my life. When actually life is meant to be lived. That simple. In fact, I just read a quote from the Dalai Lama that was on my friend's wall where I had Easter dinner and that was super inspiring about living life.

Every day, think as you wake up, today I am fortunate to be alive, I have a precious human life, I am not going to waste it. I am going to use all my energies to develop myself, to expand my heart out to others, to achieve enlightenment for the benefit of all beings. I am going to have kind thoughts towards others, I am not going to get angry or think badly about others. I am going to benefit others as much as I can.

~ Dalai Lama XIV

What I take from this quote and from my recent revelation is that it's not what I do with my life, but rather it's how I choose to live my life, the intention behind it. Being too focussed on the 'what' interferes with simply allowing myself to contribute in whatever way. I guess it comes back to the perfectionist issue, instead of waiting to be perfect, just start. Just live, share and express, and trust that from my intention whatever comes will be a gift and be of benefit. *I realize that this way of living is the Enlightenment Technique taught on Enlightenment/ Illumination Intensives: put your attention on the object of your enlightenment, intend to be in union with the truth of it, be open to whatever arises and to the truth in this moment, and express whatever arises as a result of your intention.*

One of my yoga students told me the other day that yoga has changed her life. She loves yoga and it has transformed her experience of being in her body and the way that she does things. This impact on someone's life is profound and, in itself, makes my life worthwhile. A part of me has always wanted to do something 'big' and 'meaningful' with my life, to 'make a big difference' in the world, but I realize that that was coming from ego, that part that wanted and needed to validate my existence. It doesn't mean I'm not open or willing to have a big impact or make a big difference; in fact, in some ways I already have, but I don't feel I 'need' to anymore. I have lost that ambition. If it happens organically, just from the pure and authentic expression and sharing of my heart then great—but if not, that's okay too.

APRIL 11

**The most beautiful thing we can experience
is the mysterious. Is the source of all true art and
all science. He to whom this emotion is a stranger, who can
no longer pause to wonder and stand rapt in awe,
is as good as dead: his eyes are closed.
~ Albert Einstein**

I'm doing my best to renew my conviction. I feel it growing stronger. Yesterday I rode my bike to Linnaea for a yoga class, and the ride felt really good. I was remembering how good it felt to be physical. It's funny how I can know what is good for me; in fact, in my mind I have the perfect recipe for total and complete well-being and yet I don't do it. What's stopping me? Or is it even possible to have 'the perfect recipe.' It feels too rigid. There must be a way to make positive supportive choices and not feel locked into a certain way of being. It's that ongoing dance between intention and openness, focus and flow. I suppose I am living that to a certain degree as I don't seem to get that stuck in anything anymore. I can be highly disciplined and live austerely, and I can let go of all rules and be completely indulgent. That's a pretty cool realization actually. Even exciting and liberating. Perhaps I am freer than I think I am. But is freedom really all it's made out to be? There seems to be a cost to freedom or maybe it's dependent upon what I choose to do with that freedom. Yeah, that feels right.

This feels like a very potent time for me, almost like a quickening that I've heard about. My tarot reading said I would birth something that was uniquely me the middle of this month. That's a few days away. As you know, I had thoughts that it might be this book, but that seems unlikely at this point, although not out of the realm of possibility. At any rate, I just had the thought that perhaps in line with my Easter revelation, it's not a physical, material thing—it's actually me! I feel like I am re-emerging more fully and purely as myself than ever before. Free from external or ingrained influences. I feel more and more that I am allowing myself to be in the place of mystery and curiosity, letting myself unfold newly in each moment. Not completely and totally but more than ever. I also feel myself getting closer to Spirit, the Mystery. A lot of animal presence has been in my life lately, in quite a magical way. Deer coming closer to me than ever before, hummingbirds, owls, wolf.

My friend, Erin, and I were having a Hakomi session over Skype the other day. She was telling me about Bhakti Yoga and that it's a direct link to the Divine and develops a personal connection to Spirit. That sparked something in me. I thought of my destiny card and how life's adversities are meant to drive me closer to Spirit, so why not just go straight to Spirit on my own. Choose it. Why wait for more adversity? A direct connection to Spirit is something I've been trying to establish for quite a while actually, but I guess something in me has been resisting in some way. That part of me that doubts and questions. Yet there is such a deep part of me that yearns for that connection, to trust fully. I guess I'm wary of making that connection for the wrong reason, which seems absurd as soon as I write that. But I don't want to use Spirit as a 'scapegoat.'

HAKOMI

Hakomi therapy is a form of body-centered somatic psychotherapy developed by Ron Kurtz in the 1970s and furthered by a group led by Kurtz in the 1980s. The Hakomi method combines Western psychology, systems theory and body-centered techniques with the mindfulness and non-violence principles of Eastern philosophy. Hakomi is grounded in seven principles: mindfulness, nonviolence, organicity, unity, body-mind holism, truth and mutability. ~ Wikipedia

One of my teachers once said that full surrender isn't really possible or healthy until one takes full responsibility for one's life. I'm getting there, but man, it's been a long arduous journey. So much resistance and unconscious behaviour and so many unconscious choices. One of my revelations during the Hakomi session with Erin was that I can fully claim my life as my own, which seems so obvious and absurd and yet so elusive in some weird way. The choice to live my life in total integrity with who I am and what's in my heart seems so simple and obvious and, at the same time, radical. It's scary, too, because it does mean taking full responsibility for my life, for all of my choices, my failures, my accomplishments, my current situation. They are all my doing. And I've 'known' this on some level, heard it dozens of times and yet it's just sinking in.

Then the question arises—what would I do differently? What do I want to make my life about? Thoughts of certain details about my life come to mind, things I would change, and yet I don't want to get caught up in details. I want to focus on the essence of being—how do I want to live my life? Versus—what do I want to do with my life? And yet, having said that, both seem important.

Mostly I want my life to be about love, of course, being as loving as possible. I want to be a source of contribution to others. I want all that I say and do to be of benefit to the well-being of people and the planet. I want to express myself fully and freely in a way that doesn't do harm to anyone or anything.

A voice says, "You're doing all this already."

Another voice says, "Are you nuts? Don't be such a flake."

Another voice says, "Woopty-do, doesn't everyone?"

There's a part of me that wants to let go of all of my own ideas and thoughts of how I should be and what I should be doing and fully surrender to 'God's will.' I shake my head and stick out my tongue and groan. Back to this again. This fucking dilemma of which is my will versus God's will. Is there a difference? How do I know? It's a fucking vicious cycle. Here I thought I was really getting somewhere. What a laugh. I crack myself up. You must think I'm a total nutbar.

April 19

Israel

I'm in Jerusalem with my family: dad; my second mom, Marilyn; and my brother, Jonah. It's Holocaust Memorial Day. We spent the day at the Holocaust Museum, the largest in the world. It was a deeply moving and humbling experience. I felt sick to my stomach and moved to tears within the first ten minutes. It's a national holiday that starts on the eve at 5pm. At that time, we were in the old city and had just left the Wailing Wall. As five o'clock approached, the temperature dropped significantly and a howling wind blew through the city. The sky darkened with ominous clouds, and the weather reflected the mood of the moment, as if God was letting us know he was there. At 10am on the day of Holocaust Memorial, a siren sounds, and everyone stops and stands in silence, the entire country. Even people driving their cars stop where they are, get out and stand with heads down remembering and honouring those who suffered. It was a profound moment. We were walking on the street when it happened. Our plan was to already be at the museum, but we got lost. We were meant to be on the street; it was more profound that way, seeing how the whole city just stops. It was incredibly moving to bear witness to, to be a part of, and to experience an entire nation standing together for two minutes in silence.

It made me wonder that if an entire country can stop, be still and pray, why couldn't entire continents—or even the entire world—unite to stop and take a stand for world peace. I recall a moment during a Landmark seminar in which I stood up and made the declaration that I take a stand for world peace, and most everyone in the room stood with me. If more of us did that, wouldn't it spread? While I was in the museum seeing the images of starving people, I also thought of my crazy idea that I had about a world hunger strike.

From My
Heart
To Yours

When I had this idea, my boyfriend at the time thought I was crazy and was quite disturbed by it, but I still think that it could be a viable solution or catalyst for world peace and that if enough people got on board with the mission, the world would be forced to take notice and take action. *My idea was to start a world hunger strike until all the terms of our requests were met, such as the end of all war, all toxins forbidden, the end of injustice, clean water and food for all, etc.*

So many people just stood by and allowed the Holocaust to happen. How is standing by and allowing all of the injustice that is happening in the world right now any different? How can I continue to justify going about my life knowing that thousands or probably even millions of people are suffering unnecessarily? There must be a way to stop it or, at the very least, to lessen it. It seems so obvious, so simple really. And yet, as I say that, I know it's not. In fact, I recall moments in the Holocaust Museum when I felt irritated or even angry at people for being in my way or for being loud. I recognized it and immediately shifted my thoughts, but I still had them.

No matter how hard I try to be a good person, I still have nasty thoughts. That was part of my prayer at the Wailing Wall, to release any ill thoughts toward others or myself. To find peace in my own heart and then, of course, that all beings find peace, freedom and happiness. Am I too naive? No, it's important. I need to keep having hope in humanity or perhaps I am delusional.

There does seem to be so much evil in the world. Especially when I watch TV or listen to the news, I start to become present to how the human mind can work, how sick and twisted it can be, how malicious. And yet I can't understand it. I don't understand how people can wish for or, even worse, take action against others. Why are we made that way? Why do we have that capacity? For what purpose? It was appalling to see, read about and listen to what happened during World War II. Unbelievable. It's a side of humanity I haven't wanted to really look at or accept. In fact, I've spent most of my life avoiding it. That's why I don't pay attention to the news, that's why I have never owned a TV. I find it all too disturbing, unnerving, depressing.

My family has always accused me of living in a bubble and they are right. I just thought it was better to focus on what is good, focus on what I want, but maybe it has made me too complacent. Perhaps it is better to know, to feel, to see, to hear about all of the pain, injustice, hardship that others are experiencing. Perhaps that would evoke more from me. Avoiding it hasn't seemed to help anyway. I still experienced years of depression and despair. I thought it was exposing myself to the happenings of the world that aggravated my despair and made it worse, but maybe I had it all wrong. Perhaps it would have broken the spell and impassioned me to be more proactive and take more of a stand. Perhaps it still could.

My grandmother was a survivor of the Holocaust, my dad, brother, sister and I wouldn't be alive if she hadn't had the will to survive those atrocities. I remember getting that at her funeral. I am a seed from her existence. I owe my life to her spirit and her will to live; it is my responsibility and duty to honour that. To keep her spirit alive.

When I spend time around Marilyn's family and hear all about what her sister's children are up to with their lives, I feel a bit inferior, like I have been selfish and have wasted a lot of my life away on meaningless things. I feel that I haven't done nor am doing anything too significant. I know that's not being very kind or loving to myself, but I also have to be honest with myself. That is a form of love. Take stock. What have I done? Truly? To contribute to the world? Sure, I have impacted and contributed to peoples' lives. But in any way that truly makes a lasting difference? Not to the degree that I feel satisfied with.

I can start to see why a lot of Jewish people have been so successful and have taken powerful steps to make their mark on the world. It's almost disrespectful not to. A dishonour to all those who perished and all those who survived and all that it took, all that they endured. I just don't know what I am supposed to do. How can I make more of a difference? Become a teacher? Psychotherapist? Lawyer? Start a movement? Become more political? I still do feel the call to work with youth and children, to help instill values and self-worth and passion. To inspire and educate others to care and to take an interest in the well-being of others and the planet.

Jonah thinks that my motto on my card is too weak, not specific enough: 'Dedicated to the well-being of people and the planet.' I actually feel sad that he thinks people won't take me seriously if I put that on my card. As if it's not believable or it's flaky or unrealistic. But that's truly how I feel and how I want to live my life. Why couldn't the world be run by people that actually cared?

I saw a fascinating video[16] the other day that was a spoof about the government. An alien asks a guy about the government, and the alien says something so profound and yet so simple, 'If politicians have that much power, they must be the wisest, most honest, caring and respected people on your planet." It's appalling that the answer to that is no. Inexcusable, really.

How have we stood by and let this happen? How do we just carry on with our lives and days when we know that people are being killed, that people are starving, that companies are getting away with poisoning our earth? How is it any less excusable than what happened during the holocaust? When enough of us know what is right and just, how do we just sit back and do nothing? I guess the better question is, "How do I?" Then the question arises again, "What should I do? What can I do? Does it matter, or is it simply that I hold the intention and take action in the moment and trust I will know what to do as the moment arises? Do I need a plan? No, just a mission, a vision, and begin to share it. Join forces with those that share it.

A small group of thoughtful people could change the world. Indeed, it's the only thing that ever has.
~ Margaret Mead

It's time, there can be no more excuses. It's time to stand up and take action for what I know to be right and good. Nothing less will do. That's all I need to know, the rest will come. I feel scared and nervous and excited and a little sad. Sad, perhaps, because it has taken me so long to get to this place and, even now, I question and doubt whether I will truly follow through. I have held this vision for a while, but I wasn't strong enough within myself yet. Perhaps now I am. We shall see. It is time for my life to become about something bigger than me. It's clear. Whether that's simply a family, a project, a movement ... I don't know. Time will tell. My life is unfolding as it should. There is no accident that I am here at this time. It was the perfect catalyst, a call to action, a next level of awakening. I am so grateful for all that I have, I am truly blessed and now it is time to share the blessings of my life with others. So be it.

May 3

Cortes Island

I'm back on the Island. A mix of feelings. Not liking myself very much right now. I realized that last night when I was dancing to the beat of the drums and reflecting on how I've been with people. I've been selfish, judgmental, stingy, resistant, opinionated. I'm justified in not liking myself, and I actually think it's a good thing. Being honest about how I've been acting provides an impetus to be a better person. As long as I don't let my self-loathing crush me. It's the same theme over and over again: hardship, pain, challenge. You can either let it defeat you or motivate you. It's such a thin line.

So much has happened that I've wanted to capture but have been completely unmotivated and undisciplined. I'm hoping I can recall some of the more poignant and profound moments. There have been quite a few. I thought I was inspired to write today but, as I try to get the words out, I find the energy draining out of me and that familiar feeling of dullness, heaviness slathered with self-doubt. Not sure what's going on. Has a part of me totally given up on myself? That's what it feels like. I know everything I need to do to be healthier and happier, and yet there's this huge resistance inside of me that requires massive effort to overcome. It's just easier to succumb to the resigned, and even counter, tendencies. Laziness, indulgence, procrastination, lethargy, defeatism are winning over.

MAY 4

I'm struggling. Not feeling much love for anyone, particularly myself. Feeling foggy, groggy, cranky, edgy, achy and grumpy. A few new dwarfs there! At least I still have a bit of humour. I'm not sure what's going on. I feel totally dissatisfied with my life. I didn't enjoy teaching yoga today; it felt like a bit of a grind. Feels like I'm stuck in a rut. I feel like I'm treading water. Back to doing the same old thing: bodywork, yoga and trying to keep/look busy.

I'm doubting I'll ever do anything different with my life. I'll never do the yoga video that I've been talking about for years, nor the meditation CD, nor complete this book, nor have a family. I feel that familiar fog of hopelessness and despair descending upon me and enveloping my heart and any remaining sense of inspiration. My body hurts, my head and heart are heavy, I feel alone and disconnected. I don't have any energy or motivation to do anything even though I have many things I could be doing. I need to clean my house, I could be working on my yoga video or meditation CD, I could be …

MAY 5

It's a beautiful sunny day, and I can't seem to get myself out of the house. I'm in agony, both physically and emotionally. I keep having images of taking a knife into my body to cut out the pain. All I want to do is curl into a ball and cry. Ideally in someone's arms, but no one is here to do that with. I feel really alone and pathetic. I was about to go outside to plant some seeds and something in me wouldn't let me walk out the door, so instead I've decided to write about what's going on for me.

I feel tormented and in anguish. My body tight, brow furrowed, emotion bubbling beneath the surface, my heart clenched, pressure in my head. I feel like I want to lash out and scream and kick and wail, but another part of me can barely move. I'm tired, unmotivated, and I feel like I'm barely holding on to my will to live. I know that sounds dramatic, but it's how I feel. I don't understand why I'm feeling so hopeless and sad. I have so much going for me, so much to be grateful for, and yet all I can feel and see is my deficiencies and pain. So much self-loathing. Now I'm convinced that this book is useless, just as I am. I'll never amount to anything. I'm a pathetic excuse for a human being.

Sound familiar? Where do we get this shit from? How could anyone ever say that to anyone especially themselves? Someone said that to my mom once, someone who supposedly loved her. So many injustices in the world, so much hurt, so much destruction—it's amazing what we will endure. My God, I want so desperately to be held right now so I can just cry. I don't know what to do or what's the best thing for me right now. Lie down, go for a walk, go to a friend's place, plant some seeds? I feel so disconnected from my truth and from what I need, except for what's not available—loving arms to hold me. This feeling of not being able to get what I want and feeling useless and of no good to others is where the thoughts of suicide come from. Feeling so disconnected and hopeless and useless and alone. Feeling unsure about how to get out of it, this self-imposed prison, even though I've been here so many times before and got out then, obviously. I feel stuck, locked in. I need to ask for help but not sure who to reach out to, not wanting to impose myself on anyone, not wanting to ruin anyone's day especially when it's such a beautiful sunny spring day. I don't want to be a downer.

MAY 6

It's become glaringly obvious to me that my love for myself is conditional. I withhold my love and even punish myself if I don't meet my own expectations for myself. To earn my own love and acceptance, I must eat a particular way, look a certain way, feel a certain way, interact accordingly, and have a certain degree of accomplishment and success in specific areas of life. I have all of these fabricated parameters that I must meet to qualify for self-love and acceptance. It's ridiculous. No wonder I suffer so much and want to kill myself. I am my own worst enemy. So the question is how do I shift this? I guess the first and biggest step is the awareness of it, naming it and outing myself. Then deciding that I want to change this behaviour.

Patience. That's the message I got from a dharma talk I went to tonight. It's important to have patience on this wild and wacky journey of life. I set the intention to master self-love and acceptance because I've isolated the lack of these as the main source of my suffering.

I had a thought today as I was giving a really great massage that perhaps I need to accept that that's what I am at this point in my life. I am a kick-ass bodyworker who gives a mean-ass massage. I keep talking about and thinking about how I don't want to be a bodyworker for the rest of my life, so I'm always trying to figure out what else I'm supposed to be. Instead, I could be focussing on being great at what I am doing now and trust that when I'm not meant to be doing bodywork anymore, I will know what to do or I'll figure it out then. Just be present with and grateful for the honour and privilege I have of being with and sharing with people in this way. It is quite beautiful and rewarding, and at what other job could I make $40 to $100 per hour and have semi-flexible hours. Sure it's a little challenging physically, but it motivates me to stay healthy and strong.

Yes, that's the next step for me in self-love and acceptance. Accept and love that I teach yoga and do bodywork for a living. I'm extremely blessed in fact! I realize that part of me has been embarrassed or ashamed that that's what I do for a living, like it's not 'good enough' or 'professional enough' or valid. But, in fact, it's an amazing way to make a living. I have been present to how amazing it is at times, but I don't think I have ever fully acknowledged it. I get to love people up and get paid for it. I get to guide and teach people how to love themselves. My God, woman! Wake up and smell the chai rooibos! It's incredible how hard I can get on myself, how much I think I should be other than I am. It's crazy making. This year I am dedicating myself to accepting, loving and being present with myself and my life. Being grateful and being content. For real. It's time to truly live what I know and practise what I preach. Walk my talk. No more excuses.

MAY 7

An amazing day. I went to a profound dharma talk that spoke right to my soul and heart. She talked about spiritual urgency that comes from the yearning and from the ache in our heart for meaning and understanding. 'Samvega.' Surrender with full participation. Doing nothing with 100% commitment.

SAMVEGA

Samvega was what the young Prince Siddhartha felt on his first exposure to aging, illness, and death. It's a hard word to translate because it covers such a complex range—at least three clusters of feelings at once: the oppressive sense of shock, dismay, and alienation that come with realizing the futility and meaninglessness of life as it's normally lived; a chastening sense of our own complacency and foolishness in having let ourselves live so blindly; and an anxious sense of urgency in trying to find a way out of the meaningless cycle.[17]

MAY 8

It's funny how the Universe always seems to send me clients that reflect my current life situation. My client today is working with letting go of any attachment and expectation of a partner making him happy. When I asked him if that were gone, what would that open up for him, what would become possible, he said, "Unconditional self-love."

Phenomenal. Of course, exactly what I am working on. He said he got the programming from his father, which made me look at where I possibly got the idea that I needed a partner in my life to be complete. I can see how it was from many different sides. Every family gathering, the first questions are about relationship and children: When are you getting married? When are you having a baby? It is relentless. I can see how this could cause me to think I was somehow deficient without a relationship and a family. I've been trying to determine whether having a committed relationship is truly authentic to me, and this might be a key. Sometimes it does seem like a deep truth and, other times, I'm not sure. Wondering if I'm meant to simply be a lover, sharing affection and connection when the opportunity arises. Being mother to my friends' children. I don't know.

I'm really struggling with this writing. Not enjoying it anymore. Constantly criticizing. I have these profound thoughts throughout the day and get excited to capture them in writing, and yet when I sit down to write, I can't seem to express myself in a satisfactory way. Not at all like I was when I first began. I guess it's just a phase that's reflecting the lack of self-love I am currently experiencing.

I was looking at my motto earlier on a sticker I had created a long time ago, "Love to Live, Live to Love." I've since shortened it to "Love to Live to Love" or "Live to Love to Live." Anyway, when I saw my motto, it struck me how integral it is to cultivate self-love. It's at the core of everything I do and every relationship I have. If I'm not loving myself then my life and relationships will reflect that—does reflect that. Look at my experience with writing for example. Yes, this is my life project: self-love. And this book will follow, track and capture this journey. I have always been curious to know whether it is truly possible. So why not settle the matter or at least explore it as fully as I can?

You know it's quite fascinating. It's almost as if the Universe has been conspiring for me to follow this path of exploring, cultivating and mastering self-love, and yet I have spent so much time denying and/or resisting it. Crazy. Kripalu Yoga is all about self-love and compassion. Most of the WarriorSage teachings and practices were about that. Lawrence, one of my main teachers is all about the 'pilgrimage of love.' Lomi Lomi and the Hawaiian Shamanic teachings, Huna is all about love—Aloha. *Things that make you go hmmm … ;-)*

MAY 20

**Self-study, as it's practiced even in the East,
is about reducing the unnecessary suffering
that comes from not knowing who you really are.**
~ Ron Kurtz

It's a new moon today. I read the beginning of my book last night.
I was re-inspired to start writing again. I had started it on the new
moon and, before I went to bed last night, I was wondering when
the next new moon was and saw that it was today. A sign! ;-) So here
I go again. It's raining after two weeks of solid sun. A perfect day
to stay in and rest and write but, alas, I am scheduled to give some
sessions and then perhaps play in an Ultimate Frisbee tournament.

It's been difficult to get out of bed lately. I've been feeling so tired,
I even had a headache last night. I'm not sure what it's from, I guess
it could just be that it's my moon time. Also, I assisted a week-long
yoga training that went from 7am to 10pm most days, and during
breaks I gave massages or taught yoga. So I guess you could say I've
been putting out a lot of energy. I've also been receiving a lot. The
Psoma Yoga training was phenomenal. The creator of Psoma Yoga,
Donna Martin is such a blessing, the true embodiment of all the
qualities of being I aspire to: compassionate, authentic, lighthearted,
easy going, loving, joyful, patient, real, humourous, modest, attentive,
approachable, appreciative, expressive. She's my latest superhero but
not in a way that is superior but instead inspiring and attainable. If
that makes any sense. She evokes those qualities in myself, and I get
to experience what it's like to be in a more present, accepting and
compassionate place. It's lovely, sweet, soft, open, warm, supportive
and nourishing. It's a shame they don't teach this stuff in schools.

My favourite tool that I learned from Donna, which I use on an ongoing daily basis, is to simply breathe in appreciation and breathe out love. This can be done anywhere anytime. I often do it when I'm out for a walk or sitting quietly, while washing dishes or while giving a session or even when in a line-up at the grocery store or bank. It's particularly fun out in public.

PSOMA YOGA

Yoga for self-awareness: a mindfulness-based way of integrating body, mind and spirit. This integration, or what I call remembering wholeness, is the traditional point of yoga practice. Soma refers to the body, ps (as in psyche) refers to mind and spirit ... hence the term I coined: Psoma Yoga. It is this integrative approach to yoga, practiced in mindful awareness for self-understanding, healing, compassion and liberation. ~ Donna Martin

I just got home from the Ultimate party, and I'm the most drunk I've been in a long time. I didn't even drink that much. I'm aware of the part of me that won't let go of control. It's so rare that I actually let myself go completely. I'm not sure what I'm afraid of. In some way I think it's a good thing that I'm wanting to stay conscious and be conscious of my actions. I think it's a really good thing. I'm not even sure why I drank as much as I did, except that I was probably trying to numb some feelings of neglect and loss.

The man I was dating a while back was there, and I felt a little ignored and avoided all night. The one time we did connect it was fleeting and felt strained and awkward. I'm concerned that I scared him away with my intensity when we were dating and part of me feels like I wasn't even given a chance. I think I'm taking it all too personally; he told me he needed time for himself to heal and grow stronger. I wonder if he was totally telling the truth though. I guess I could ask him. I'm not sure why it matters. I guess I'm wondering whether I should completely let go and I'm thinking I should. I'm not sure if he's right for me anyway. I actually don't have a clue what's right for me. I think I have some ideas, but I could be so off base.

I do know that I want a man who is loving, caring, honest, respectful, aware, conscious, funny, family oriented, passionate, playful, adventurous, patient, kind, understanding, sensual, affectionate, strong, open minded, resourceful, integral, supportive, creative … I think those are the essentials, any details beyond that are a bonus. I'm willing to be surprised—pleasantly, I hope. Part of me wonders if I deserve such a good man, and the other part of me is, "Of course! You're amazing." Part of me was thinking that I should hide away from men completely until I at least finish this book or succeed at something. Why would any man want to be with a woman in debt?!

I don't know why or how I came to be so hard on myself. A lot of women are in debt who find a great man. My first husband helped me to pay off my student loans when we lived and worked in Japan. Why do I make my financial situation such a determining factor as to whether I'll find my 'soul mate' or not?! I wonder what will become of me? Will I die a lonely old maid? Will I connect and share my life with my soul mate? Will I become a mother? Will I make or inherit a fortune or die a pauper? Am I meant to be a monk? Will I ever finish this book? If so, will anyone ever read it? I almost feel like I need to take a month or so out just to dedicate to writing. Life is too distracting. When life is happening, I just want to be in it and am usually too tired or worn out to write. So much has happened that I want to share. But I get so caught up in time: there's not enough time, I need to go to bed to get some sleep, and I'll have time tomorrow. So many excuses.

I've been letting myself down a lot lately, haven't kept up with my commitments to myself. It's time to recommit, and yet I've been having a great life. That's the ongoing dance, trying to find the balance between structure and flow. I suspect that if I did some more of the things that are good for me that I would have more energy, ease and flow. "Consciousness loves contrast," as dear Donna Martin would say. I have to experience what it's like to live not doing the things that nourish and support me so then, when I do do them, I can really get the power and impact and can perhaps recommit with more fervour and joy. Who knows. It did feel good to do Yoga Nidra today, dance a little, do some yoga and write. Yep. Make my life about what's important and what brings me joy! Keep remembering!

I think I'm doing pretty damn good. Not much to complain about. Life is very sweet, and I feel completely and utterly blessed. Hmmm, makes me wonder if I have any new moon intentions ... to plant my garden and keep nurturing the seeds I've already planted such as this book, my friendships, family ties, my work, my community, my health and well-being, creativity and connection to spirit. It's a good life, and I am oh so grateful.

MAY 21

I'm writing with resistance. I almost just went to bed, and then I thought better of it. Keep up my commitment, recommitment to myself. I just don't know what to write about. I guess that's the point, I don't have to know. Just start writing and see what comes.

I just read some fascinating stuff from Stephen Cope's book. He was talking about the importance and even necessity of both awareness and equanimity. If you have one without the other, imbalance happens that can result in fragmentation. I think that's what happened to me, why I went a little crazy after my first Enlightenment/Illumination Intensive. He said that too much awareness without—what does he call it?—the "abiding self" overloads the system, and we crash basically. He says it so much better:

> When equanimity is weak there will be increasing fragmentation. When awareness is weak, we'll find ourselves constantly hijacked by our unconscious projects. As more abiding center is cultivated, it calls for and creates the container for more awareness. As awareness is honed, and more of the unconscious is revealed, it calls for a stronger abiding center to hold it.[18]

I think that's why I'm so in love with Psoma Yoga—it is all about this balance. Cope also talks about the importance of including the body, which is a big piece of the Psoma Yoga that was missing in my previous modalities for helping others. It's just a way better fit for me being such a 'body-oriented' person. I'm grateful for all the learning and skills I gained from my previous practices. They are a great foundation for the Psoma Yoga work. I can see why I never really got a practice going. It just wasn't the right fit for me. My heart wasn't fully in it. I can honestly and enthusiastically say that my whole heart and soul is in Psoma Yoga. It's the perfect fit. I'm curious where I'll go with it. I'd like to talk to Donna about the possibilities. Whether I should just develop my own style of practice or get sanctioned under her and, as I write this, the answer is obvious to me. My own style. It's time to own who I am and own that I have unique gifts to offer that will serve others. I was getting this on a deeper level during the Quantum Light Breath Meditation tonight, this sense of being authentically and uniquely expressed, which comes from owning and putting my whole self in my expression.

MAY 22

It's late and I want to go to bed, but I also want to keep up the momentum and maintain my renewed commitment to myself and to writing. I had a really great day: cleaned house; visited my friend, Monika; sat in the sun with her and her kids watching the hens and roosters; gave a beautiful session; watered my garden; cycled to Hollyhock for a presenter evening on Core Energetics; and was reminded of the power of vulnerability and authenticity. Was reunited with an old friend, had a good boogie and was told by a woman who I've never met that my dancing brought her joy. I cycled home in the dark under the stars, listening to the croaking of the frogs and felt so good to be alive. It is a truly blessed life I have.

It's funny—I have a male friend coming to visit, someone that my second mom thinks is my soul mate. When I let her know by text that he was coming to visit, she sent me a message telling me that I should get some therapy to work through my issues before he comes. I sent a snarky message back even though I knew she was joking, but—oddly enough—tonight in the lodge after the presenter evening, a few of us were having tea and did a process that works through the blocks around getting what we want. I worked on, "I want a relationship." It was pretty fascinating. My friend pretended to be me and said over and over, "I want a relationship." And I replied with whatever reasons or excuses I have as to why I can't have one. At one point, my mind was blank, and I could sense the real possibility of having a relationship. It was tangible and powerful. It's a great way to flush out our unconscious counter intentions and test whether we really want what we think we want. It felt like I was purifying my intention.

I feel like I'm being and living more and more authentically all the time, and it feels really good. Right. Healthy, wholesome. There's so much I want to share but feel the call to bed more strongly. I need to carve out a specific chunk of time just for writing. I'll do that.

From My
Heart
To Yours

MAY 23

I'm listening to my radio show from last week and I'm impressed. It actually sounds really good. I love what I'm saying and how it flows with the choice of songs. Powerful messages and super inspiring. I'm blown away by myself. ;-) I'm obviously feeling really good about myself and my life right now. I had this moment while dancing to the live drums at the hall where I could feel myself opening up to living more freely and fully, being more 'me.'

I planted more seeds today! I have a garden! You have no idea how thrilling that is for me. I had this moment in the garden after a lot of weeding and shoveling where I felt this joy bubble up in me; there's nothing like hands in the dirt! My dreams truly are all coming true. It's so amazing. So many simple yet magical moments throughout the day. The deer grazing in my yard who doesn't move when I pull up, 'radiant being' shouted out to me from a beautiful tree-limbing man, and having the honour of being part of people's healing/life journey. So many magical moments.

MAY 24

Hmmm … I'm stuck for words. I'm really tired and have a low-grade headache. My friend 'Duncan' (his pseudonym) is here, he came to visit. He's a friend from Edmonton, someone I've known for about twenty years. The one my second mom thinks is meant to be my man. We're having a nice visit. There's an ease, laughter, kindness, respect. I'm curious and open. I did Qi Gong this morning, I love it. I need to do it more often. I feel like I'm not tapping into and accessing the energy that's available to me. I've been feeling tired, weak and fatigued like I would at the end of the season, and the season is just beginning. Something feels out of whack. Maybe I just need to do a cleanse.

I talked to a friend who's expecting to die in a few weeks or months. He contacted me to tell me he was dying, so that I could be a source of support for his daughter. She was a participant in an Illumination Intensive I once co-facilitated, and we had a special bond. He and I had a wild conversation. He's actually excited about death, more excited than he was about life. In fact, he's looking forward to it. He finds life quite difficult and painful, and he just wants to get out. He had an experience at an Illumination Intensive in which he said he crossed the veil and experienced the most divine love and acceptance, and he wants more of that. Who can blame him? Why is this life so challenging and painful, so full of suffering? I agree with him when he says that things in this world are all backwards and don't make sense. Like the fact that the people who are creating the most destruction and harm on the planet get paid the most money and the people who are providing nurturing, love and inspiration get paid the least or not at all. Sometimes I feel guilty for what feels kind of like 'opting out' by living here *(on a remote island)* and for not engaging in the rat race and crazy game/system that's been created. But I don't agree with it, so why participate? I have to live in integrity with what's in my heart.

MAY 27

Wow, how quickly things can change. I'm in love, totally utterly smitten. Have met my soul mate, well—discovered that someone I've known for twenty years is my soul mate. The connection between us is profound. When I'm with him, when he looks at me, when he touches me, my insides are ignited. I feel bliss in his arms. There's a deep and clear knowing that we are meant to be together, we both feel it. Our connection just feels so right, so natural, so real. Last night, we both dreamt of each other. This morning we were telling each other about our dreams. He dreamt that he asked me if I would give him a child, and that gave me the courage to tell him I had dreamt that I told him I was falling in love with him. We opened right up to each other and started planning our future together.

There was no discussion of whether this was right or of how we really feel, how can we really know. There was just a clear and understood knowing that we are meant to be together. Exactly and yet beyond what I imagined. He asked if he could make all my dreams come true, and he asked me if I would give him a child, and I said, "Yes, yes, yes!" I had a 'yes' as soon as he told me about his dream; in fact, I had a 'yes' on the second night we were together. The deciding moment was probably when he was helping me plan my radio show by suggesting songs to use, and he put on Vera Lynn, "As Time Goes By." And I was thinking how I'd love to dance, and he looked down at me and asked me if I wanted to dance. I said an emphatic, "Yes!" I got up and he asked if he had just read my mind, and I said, 'Yes!' Then we danced into total blissdom. I completely lost myself in his arms, felt so much incredible energy moving through my body, into my heart. I kept thinking about Oriane Lee's (the tarot reader) advice to pay attention to my energy around different men, and my energy around Duncan was off the charts.

From My
Heart
To Yours

We have no idea how we're going to be together, but we trust we'll find a way: him living in Edmonton and me here on Cortes. We agreed to take it one day at a time. So much sweetness, tenderness, care and love was shared between us. And we also had some fun adventures and intelligent discussions. He fulfilled all my hopes in a man, telling me I look beautiful, conscientious, telling me he adores me, massaging me, dancing with me, respectful, generous, considerate, appreciative, the way he held me firmly yet tenderly, the way he would hold my gaze, humour, honesty. I felt so happy and giddy, and yet not in an immature, fantasy way. It felt like divine providence brought us together, like destiny.

I know I'm sounding corny and verging on ridiculous, but I can't explain how right and real our connection was/is. There's no doubt or second guessing or questioning. Just pure true knowing that we are meant to share our lives together and that our life will be magical and real and good. At one point he said, "This is good, isn't it?" And indeed it is. This is good. Really truly good.

MAY 30

It's 3am. I woke up to go pee, and now I can't get back to sleep. Not sure why. It could be all the dark chocolate I ate at my friend's faery birthday party, or it could be my aching heart. I never imagined I'd be in a long distance relationship. It's tortuous. I thought the knowing that I had finally found my soul mate would provide a lasting peace and joy, but that faded within twenty-four hours. I basked in the glow of our connection for the first day or so. Now all I feel is the anguish of our separation and longing to be reunited. And, of course, the mind and all its tricky ways are bringing in doubt and questioning: Is this real? Will this last? Will he change his mind? We don't really even know each other. We're too different. It's too good to be true. I'm not good enough for him. And on and on it goes …

But underneath all that is the solid and clear knowing that we are meant to be together. The sweetness that we shared, the care, the tenderness, the love is indisputable and everlasting. And maybe you'll think that's faery tale, but in my heart of hearts I know it to be true. At least it's inspired me to write! ;-)

Insecurities are such a funny thing. Oh, I'm just remembering a dream I had about me and the local youth. I came into a room where they all were and, as I entered, I saw most of them look at me and then turn to each other and whisper things. Then the others turned and looked, so I knew they were talking about me. I assumed it was something mean or nasty. I had the choice to shy away and ignore them, but instead I chose to go up to them and talk to them. I told them that I felt awkward around them and that I got all insecure when I was with them, but I wanted them to know how amazing I thought they were and that I really liked them. Then they all changed, or at least I perceived them to change, and their faces became all sweet and soft and accepting. They smiled and laughed and everything was good between us. I know the awkwardness I feel is my own stuff, and I need/want to work through it. Some of them may very well judge me, but I can't let that get in the way of seeing them for who they are. I feel like I revert back to that insecure little girl when I'm around them, it's so strange.

I used to think I wanted to be a teacher, but I don't think I do. I want to be a mother. What else I'm meant to do, I'm not sure. I do want to keep expanding my capacity to help people and be a source of contribution to others, but I'm not sure in what way. I've been thinking a lot more about getting my master's, so I could be more legit and be a counsellor of some sort. But maybe I don't need it. I should just start offering yoga therapy sessions and see what happens. I also want to expand my coaching business.

I can't understand what's getting in the way of getting more clients. I've seen profound and rapid results with my one friend who I've been coaching, and it's only been a few weeks—and thirty minutes a week at that. Just start! Remember! That's the message of this book at the very beginning. I don't have to have it all figured out, just start and see where it goes from there. One person at a time and let it build organically. That's what Duncan and I said about our relationship when we started to look at and plan how we'd form our future together, one day at a time. Otherwise it becomes too overwhelming and seemingly impossible.

I feel good to be writing again. I know I have good and important things to share. Real life stuff. And I know and trust that it's the open and honest way that I'm willing to share that will serve you in some way or, at the very least, amuse you. I think I've said that before. But my hope is that it does help in some way, if just to let you know that you're not alone in the challenges you face in your life. Perhaps to give you hope that dreams can actually come true. To reignite your belief in the power of love. That you can live a life that you imagine is possible. You can be happy. Suffering is optional, remember?! A certain degree of suffering is optional indeed, perhaps all of it, once one becomes conscious that they are the source of their own suffering. As Donna Martin says there is a lot of unnecessary suffering that we can help alleviate. That's what I'm interested in. I gather that's one of the reasons I've experienced so much of it and worked through most of it—so that I can be a living example of what's possible. To have the compassion and knowledge that suffering happens and that it can be avoided.

"So how does one do that?" you may be asking.

Through awareness and choice. Awareness and choice result in freedom. My mind is the source of most of my suffering. My preferences, aversions, expectations, attachments, ideas, concepts, judgments, perceptions all get in the way of what's real and true. What's possible without all of these nasties in the way? Love, acceptance, compassion, grace, peace and connection. I know because I've experienced it. It's what I've witnessed in the hundreds of people who I've seen wake up at Enlightenment/ Illumination Intensives.

My mind comes in and wonders if this perspective is all my preference and preferred point of view. Good question. Possibly. I think I shared this with you already; one of my 'revelations' was that I can't 'know' anything for sure. Maybe what I've just shared is true, but maybe it's not. All I know is that it keeps coming back to love. And when I feel it, allow it, am it—when I am love—all is good in my world. It's beyond good, it's exquisite and sweet and true. Heck, if I am going to have a point of view why not take one that feels really, really good! ;-) Not only to myself but to everyone else around me. Okay, on that note, I'm going to be loving to myself and go back to bed. I'm glad I got up and did this. I could have stayed in bed and suffered, but I listened to the voice that said to get up and write. I'm happy I did. I hope you are too. ;-)

June 4

It's the full moon tonight. I guess my writing is meant to flow with the moon cycles. The full moon is a time to reflect on what we are grateful for. I certainly have a lot to be grateful for, and yet I've been feeling kind of blue, sad and melancholy. Theda mentioned the other day that I might be slightly bi-polar. It's certainly possible. I have had my share of mood swings, highest of the highs to lowest of the lows. But another friend thinks it's natural. I think there might be some sort of chemical imbalance. What else would explain the unjustified bouts of sadness I constantly go through? Although I was reflecting earlier that it's been 14 months since I hit total despair. That's pretty big. I guess it's natural and even understandable that I'm feeling a little down. I've hardly been working, my beloved is over a thousand kilometres away, it's been a bit grey and cool outside, I'm feeling lonely and a little bored. My energy has been super low, too. Such little motivation to get the simplest things done, although I have been putting out a lot of energy. The radio show, the event I organized last weekend, hosting dinners for friends. I think it's becoming clear that I'm hard on myself, expect a lot, so rarely satisfied. I am getting better, but I do fall back to that pattern of over achievement, high expectations, impatience, and I-want-it-all-now mentality.

I was thinking while I was in the bath that it's quite perfect that Duncan lives far away. It's like the Universe has finally fulfilled that last longing so now I can stop looking, but I have the time and space to cultivate my self-love. With him being so far away, I can see those parts of me that still attach my happiness to somebody or something else. Now I can clearly see that and cultivate self-fulfillment and happiness. I guess I expected more relief from not having to look any more.

My friend said something really sweet when I told her I had met my soul mate. She said, "I feel the Universe at peace now that you have found your twin flame." So sweet, so true. And yet, this ache … for what? Why? To be with him, to start to co-create our lives together. When I think back to how I felt in his presence, I feel a bit of fear of my attachment. He just awakened so much in me and brought out so much love and tenderness—why wouldn't I want to feel that all the time? But a-ha, there's the rub, the preference … the attachment! Eek! I must enjoy all the spaces I move through, relish this time alone while I have it. I need to meditate more. I keep saying that, but I don't do it. Why do I find it so difficult to commit to the things that I know are good for me? I also need to do more yoga—daily yoga, in fact. I've been eating better, that feels good. I want to do a cleanse soon. I was thinking I will when Rachel, my new roommate, moves in, and then I can use her juicer and do a juice cleanse.

I wonder if I'll actually move back to Edmonton. I really don't want to, but part of me is willing to do it temporarily for Duncan, for us. It would be really sad to leave Cortes, and yet lately I haven't been feeling as attached to it. I feel like I don't really have many friends here. The only people I'm really close to are Monika and her kids and, yes, I would miss them dearly. In a perfect world, we would live here part time and in Victoria or Edmonton part time. Well, actually, in a truly perfect world, we would live on Cortes for the summer and somewhere tropical for the winter. It'll be interesting to see how life unfolds.

I wonder if it is crazy to think/expect that Duncan and I are meant to spend our lives together. We do barely know each other, and yet it was so crystal clear to both of us. But I've been 'crystal clear' about other things before and they didn't pan out. I still lack some trust in myself and in the Universe, I guess. The most important thing is that I'm curious and intrigued as to how it will all work out. I'm wary of things moving a little too fast, of missing out on—I don't know—some of the sweet things about courting, I guess. I want to feel romanced, I suspect he's a romancing type—but who knows? He does continue to amaze me. He's so brilliant, has such a vast array of knowledge about so many things. So different from me; I like and appreciate the differences. I have this hunger to know him, to be known by him, completely and fully—which is impossible, but as much as is possible—and to keep discovering who each other is. Yes, my heart aches to be close to him and that's okay; in fact, it's good. It's quite fascinating, the longing hasn't changed, I still long for my beloved, but now I at least know his face.

JUNE 5

It's Venus Transit right now, a time when Venus crosses the sun. I just looked at pictures of the little black dot against the sun. The next one won't be until 2117, it's a rare occurrence. An auspicious time. Supposedly, an intense time. There was just a lunar eclipse full moon last night as well. I don't know if it's due to all of this astrological stuff but, man, have I been feeling weird. Today was basically a write-off, I could barely function. I felt so out of sorts, lost, sad, confused.

I made an appointment to get a massage from Leslie, one of the Hollyhock bodyworkers. By the time I arrived to the bodywork studio, I was a mess, burst into tears, and sobbed in her arms for a good five minutes or so. Then I felt better, having that release. She asked what kind of session I wanted, and I told her nurturing, centring, balancing and TLC. I also wanted to create space and acceptance to move through whatever was going on with me. It was good. Her presence is very calming and soothing, and she's very gentle. I was able to settle more into myself and felt much better after.

I went and meditated in the Sanctuary afterward to anchor the feeling of calm and acceptance. It was right in the middle of the transit by then, supposedly a good time to meditate. I put a lot of intention today into cultivating a conscious, clear, centred, loving, compassionate, accepting, trusting, kind, gentle space for myself and my life.

I guess I'm feeling a little confused and a kind of uprooting having connected with Duncan and facing the possibility of moving again just when I thought I had found my place, my community, my home. I find myself even creating reasons to leave in my mind: I barely have any friends here anyway, nobody really calls me or invites me to anything here anyway, the island is changing, not enough people are interested in celebration or dancing here, I don't feel supported … blah blah blah.

It's amazing how quickly one's perspective can change. I don't know what's going to happen. I don't have to know. Just keep being curious and being willing to flow with what wants to happen. I do know that at this point I want to be with Duncan, and I guess my psyche is exploring whether I'm willing to move away from my discovered paradise to do that. We had a Skype date tonight after we worked out some technical kinks. He makes me laugh a lot. I'm smiling just thinking about him. Life is so fascinating. Who would have thought I'd end up connecting with a man from Edmonton, one I've known for twenty years to boot? Fascinating indeed. We'll see how it all unfolds.

JUNE 10

Well, how quickly the tables turn. Fucking hilarious, life's cruel joke. So he goes from wanting me to be the mother of his children to suggesting we be pen pals! Even after I said I'd be willing to move to Edmonton in the fall. I'm livid. I got off the phone with him, had a huge cry, needed to scream so I ran outside jumped on my bike and rode as hard as I could to the maple tree path. I screamed along the way. Walked like a mad woman down the path, got to the ocean, tore my clothes off and jumped in the ocean. It felt amazing!

I sat there for a while marvelling at the whole absurdity of the situation. Thinking how naïve and stupid I am, so caught up in the faery tale of true love. And yet part of me believes we'll get through this, it's just a test. But, man, was/am I pissed. All these things that I wanted to say to him came rushing in when I was down at the ocean. I gave space for it all, all the emotions, thoughts, sensations. Yelled a little more, cried a little more, even laughed at one point. What was it I laughed at? Oh yeah, when I realized I had just done a mini-triathlon. Biked, ran and swam. It was a cute moment, you probably needed to be there.

Anyway, I made my way home in a fury, went straight to the phone and told his answering machine exactly what was on my mind. The way I thought it was fucked that he go from asking me to be the mother of his children to being pen pals. I told him I wondered if he'd professed his devotion to any other women and then changed his mind, and said that I hoped not and that he better not do it again because it was insensitive, irresponsible and cruel. There was more. I held nothing back. It felt good. I then drew a hot bath with Epsom salts, three kinds of essential oil, made myself a cup of tension tamer tea, put on Shimshai and soaked. I guess I wasn't done because, while I soaked, I drafted an email in my head. Got out, wrote it and sent it. Told him I'd play by his rules—meaning 'write.' I have no idea how

From My
Heart
To Yours

it'll all turn out. He could meet me or pull away even more. We'll see, time will tell. I sent him *The Invitation* by Oriah Mountain Dreamer. It pretty much epitomizes the essence of a meaningful relationship, in my mind.

The Invitation

It doesn't interest me what you do for a living
I want to know what you ache for
and if you dare to dream of meeting your heart's longing.

It doesn't interest me how old you are
I want to know if you will risk looking like a fool
for love
for your dreams
for the adventure of being alive.

It doesn't interest me what planets are squaring your moon
...
I want to know if you have touched the center of your own
sorrow
if you have been opened by life's betrayals
or have become shrivelled and closed
from fear of further pain.

I want to know if you can sit with pain
mine or your own
without moving to hide it
or fade it
or fix it.

I want to know if you can be with joy
mine or your own
if you can dance with wildness
and let the ecstasy fill you to the tips of your
fingers and toes
without cautioning us to
be careful
be realistic
to remember the limitations of being human.

It doesn't interest me if the story you are telling me
is true.
I want to know if you can
disappoint another
to be true to yourself.

If you can bear the accusation of betrayal
and not betray your own soul.
If you can be faithless
and therefore trustworthy.
I want to know if you can see Beauty
even when it is not pretty
every day.
And if you can source your own life
from its presence.

I want to know if you can live with failure
yours and mine
and still stand on the edge of the lake
and shout to the silver of the full moon,
"Yes."

It doesn't interest me
to know where you live or how much money you have.
I want to know if you can get up
after a night of grief and despair
weary and bruised to the bone
and do what needs to be done
to feed the children.

It doesn't interest me who you know
or how you came to be here.
I want to know if you will stand
in the center of the fire
with me
and not shrink back.

It doesn't interest me where or what or with whom
you have studied.
I want to know what sustains you
from the inside
when all else falls away.
I want to know if you can be alone
with yourself
and if you truly like the company you keep
in the empty moments.

~ Oriah Mountain Dreamer

I guess I decided at a young age that life was cruel. In grade four,
I was in a serious car accident that scarred me for life, in more ways
than one. I received a serious gash in my face just below my left eye.
I was lucky I didn't lose my eye. My mom said the gash was so big
you could stick your finger in it. I don't remember any of it. I went
unconscious. I don't remember how long I stayed home from school

to heal, but all I remember is that when I went back, I was ostracized. Was called *The Exorcist*, the movie had just come out. I was left at the fence of the playground with no one to play with, looking on at the other children playing. I was alone. This is one of my core wounds. This is why I struggle with aloneness, separateness, despair.

It didn't start there, though. When I was five my dad left and, when I was six, my mom went into the hospital for cancer treatment in Edmonton, which was five hours away from where I lived. My aunt and uncle, with their infant son, came to look after me. I felt abandoned.

I don't remember much from my childhood. Some of my stronger memories are not pleasant. Not having anyone come to my show and tell when I was in grade one. Being pinned down by the nanny goat for what seemed like hours without any help, being chased and pecked by the rooster. Falling into the pond and almost drowning until someone did pull me out. Children teasing me about my hair, about my scar. Lots of feelings of being different and alone and unimportant. These are the themes that play over and over again in my life, in my relationships. The challenges that force me closer to God, even though I get angry with him for being so cruel; I also seek solace in her, seek guidance, understanding, meaning. I've barely slept, I woke up just after one and haven't been able to go back to sleep; it's now 4:40am. The birds started singing like crazy about twenty minutes ago so I decided to get up and write. I spent most of the time meditating and doing my best to relax, but I'm pretty wound up obviously. My head and body hurt.

This is my note from the Universe today:

For every setback, disappointment and heartbreak, Shaeah, ask yourself, "What does this create the opportunity for?" And therein you will find its gift. Everything has a reason, And if you look close enough, Shaeah, that reason will always be love, healing, or happy dancing, if not all three.
~ The Universe

From My
Heart
To Yours

Hilarious! Yes, the opportunity indeed. I guess that's why I'm writing to work it out, to gain clarity, to share my process. I am curious what this is all about. How it will all turn out. Wow, I'm soooo hungry. I already ate a muffin a few hours ago when I got up the first time. My body is so unhappy right now. I think I've done quite good considering. I spent most of the time when I was lying in bed, focussing on my breath. I even did Nadi Shodhana for quite a while.

NADI SHODHANA
Alternate Nostril Breathing

A beautiful breathing technique that helps keep the mind calm, happy and peaceful. A few minutes of Nadi Shodhan pranayama in a day is best to de-stress the mind and release accumulated tension and fatigue. The breathing technique is named *Nadi Shodhan*, as it helps clear out blocked energy channels in the body, which in turn calms the mind.

(*nadi* = subtle energy channel; *shodhan* = cleaning, purification; *pranayama* = breathing technique)[19]

I listened to the sleep meditation CD and counted my breaths. It all has served to keep me calm but not enough to shut off my brain to sleep. Oh well. It's a slow week at work. All the programs were cancelled, and there are only a few guests. It would probably be better if it was busy though, to take my mind off things but, alas, I will be forced to face this. The opportunity for healing, right? Perhaps even love and, if I'm lucky, happy dancing. There is the next Dancerama scheduled for this Friday. Five days to process and break-through, hopefully it'll be sooner than that.

Core wounds, such buggers. I had a session with Anjali the other day when I was having a tough time, and she pointed out how these childhood wounds and our beliefs that were formed by them create how we experience life. It's like a blueprint for what we can experience, and it forms our very own Universe. So if I believe that life is cruel, that I'm not important, that I'm alone then that's how I will continue to experience life. And so it is: relentless, unwavering, unforgiving. The key is to gain awareness of these unconsciously held beliefs and then with the consciousness comes choice and freedom. The opportunity to break out of the role of victim and into one of conscious choice.

At a young age, I was imprinted with a lot of disappointment, upset, hurt, cruelty, neglect and a lot of suffering and, hence, no matter how great my life seems to get, these feelings continue to haunt me and overshadow any seeming hope of happiness or fulfillment. Any time my life seems to get 'good' and I start to experience any form of contentment or happiness, it is inevitably shattered, over and over again. It's become predictable. I remember at the beginning of my connection with Duncan having the thought, "This is too good to be true." And sure enough I fulfilled my prediction. Life is fascinating. We are powerful. I guess thoughts do form our reality, to a degree. I still believe in the mystery factor. How will it all unfold? Only time will tell.

I feel the need to speak to the negative slant of my childhood that I have been portraying here. I want to make it clear that due to my state of mind at the time of writing this section, I was only seeing the negative and challenging experiences of my childhood. In actuality, I have a lot of beautiful and sweet memories and experiences from when I was young. My parents did the best that they could do, and I am grateful to them for all that I have. I love them dearly.

June 12

Forty-eight hours, one phone message, two texts, three emails and still no word from him. It's fascinating to observe my process through it all. Lots of insights from the help of others, outside perspective and some from my own inner reflection. I've learned that if I hadn't taken it so personally and hadn't reacted, I could have come more from a place of compassion and been curious about what was going on in his world to cause the shift in him. I could have given more space and time for him to process and for me to not take it on, not buy into his mind stuff. I could have been sensitive to the possibility that he just got scared and overwhelmed and, again, given him space to move through that without reacting.

It was probably naïve and foolish of me to get so caught up in the faery tale nature of our connection, we should have taken time to get to know each better before making any huge professions of love or devotion. I guess I wanted to believe in it so badly. But I really don't know him, and he doesn't know me. Someone told me today that trust builds over time, getting to know someone takes years. But having just written that, I think, "That's one person's opinion and I know of people who have met, fell in love, got married and created a family in short timespans and have stayed the test of time."

Big sigh. I don't know. Part of me is wondering if I'm supposed to take this as a wake-up call from my deluded faery tale fantasies of true love or as a test to my faith and commitment to the possibility of true love. Of course, I lean toward the latter, but I also want to be realistic and not keep making the same mistakes and keep getting hurt and disappointed. I don't know what to think or do.

At one point today, I was looking out at the trees and reflecting on the whole situation and felt totally at peace with being in a place of 'not knowing.' In fact, I felt so free and clear and good to not be attached to any particular outcome. I don't feel attached to it working out with Duncan anymore, I don't feel attached to being on Cortes for the rest of my life, I don't feel attached to needing to do anything really. I feel a deep space of acceptance and trust has opened up in me that's quite refreshing and welcome. I love where I'm at, what I'm doing, who I'm doing it with. I'm grateful for all that I have, and I trust that good things will continue to open up for me because I'm a good person with good intentions who lives, expresses and acts from my heart. I'm actually quite impressed with myself and how I'm handling the whole situation. I thought for sure I would be devastated, immobilized and in total despair for days or even weeks over this, but instead I feel clear, functional, mindful, present, curious and responsible. I'm taking good care of myself, being authentic yet not dramatic with my sharing, asking for support when I need it and have gotten to a curious and open place within a very short time.

JUNE 14

I don't think there's anything worse than heartbreak and rejection. At first I was thinking the loss of a loved one would be worse, but not even that because death is somehow more acceptable than rejection. It's not as personal. Rejection is the intentional, conscious (or maybe not so conscious) pulling away of one's love, and that really hurts. It's super hard to not take it personally. To not wonder what's wrong with me. Why am I not loveable, what did I do wrong, will I ever get it right?

I've been all over the place: sometimes okay, trusting and accepting. At other times, hitting total despair. I even started having suicidal thoughts again. I've come to the conclusion that shooting oneself is the easiest and quickest way to go; the difficult part is getting a gun. I was thinking that two guns would be the ideal, one aimed at the heart and one at the head so that way instant death is guaranteed. Don't think that's going to happen. So, the second option is jumping off the ferry weighted down with lots of heavy rocks. But the thought of the cold and the struggle doesn't appeal to me. I hate that the actions of someone else have affected me so much, that I'm so weak as to be thrown into despair by another's choice to withdraw their love from me. I don't know how to be detached. If I stop caring what other people think and stop wanting the love of another, life seems to become empty and meaningless. So what's the point?

I remember during the Landmark Forum, I had a revelatory moment of liberation when I got that life was empty and meaningless, but I don't feel that now. I just feel the loss and despair of lost dreams, hopes, desires, even innocence. I just see a life of pain, misery and loneliness because I see that anything I choose to love and connect with will someday be gone. So life is truly suffering without detachment, and I don't know how to do that. I am guaranteed a life full of disappointment, let down, loss and grief. Sure, there's the perspective of appreciating what I have in each moment, 'loving what is' as Byron Katie says, but I don't know how to sustain that in the face of loss and disappointment. And I don't know how to avoid those feelings without detachment, and I don't know how to detach.

I've been praying, doing ho'oponopono, spending time with sisters, talking about my feelings with friends and family, going for walks in nature, getting bodywork, having baths with candles, meditating, doing yoga and Qi Gong, breathing deeply, asking for support, being transparent and not hiding my feelings, writing, doing chocolate therapy, crying, giving sessions ... none of it makes the pain go away or, if it does, it's just temporary. I feel like I can't really trust anything or anyone because nothing lasts, people don't honour their word, people change their minds, people only really care about themselves (including myself).

HO'OPONOPONO

Ho'oponopono means to make things right—to correct wrongs with your relationships, including yourself. It is a beautiful process of clearing and forgiving that can set your free from many troubles, past regrets, problems with people in your life, sorrows you carry around and negativity you maintain with yourself. Ho'oponopono is a Huna technique. Huna is a very ancient system of knowledge that dates back thousands of years, to some of the earliest teachings we know of on Earth. For years it remained a secret, and as such the teachings have been kept very pure. Today, Huna teachings are available for everyone's benefit, one of the most beneficial being the teachings of Ho'oponopono.[20]

I had a realization this morning during my yoga practice when I was reflecting on and processing the whole situation with Duncan. I thought about how he has been unforgiving, uncompassionate and non-communicative. It hit me like a brick that that's exactly

From My
ℋeart
To Yours

how I've been with my friend, Zyla. It was a huge wake up call. I called her right away, explained my realization and apologized on her voicemail. I haven't heard back from her yet, but it felt good to finally own up to that. I don't even know what I've been holding on to about the whole situation, just being stubborn and righteous. Overall, I've found this whole experience to be quite humbling, to say the least.

I'm feeling very self-destructive right now. Visions of getting wasted. Images of knives and of cutting myself up. I think I must be mentally ill and emotionally unstable. Probably have been most of my life and have just done a really great job at covering it up. No wonder I'm still alone. Who would want to be with someone who's so fucked up? Although there are stories of a lot of whacked out people who were in love, crazed artists, musicians, authors, how and why did they find love and not me?

I keep having images of that big sharp knife I bought and cutting myself up, ripping myself to shreds, my arms, by stomach, my chest. I feel such despair, and I don't know who to call, who I can talk to about this? This book is the only thing keeping me alive right now, the outlet for these thoughts and feelings, the only thing preventing me from acting on my impulse to destroy my surroundings and myself. Please, God, help me to hold on. I don't know if I have the strength on my own. So much pain, I can hardly bear it. I feel so alone ....I'm barely holding on, the force so strong I tried to rip myself apart, literally. Digging finger nails into my flesh. I've called for help, it's on its way. The knife so close, a demon inside of me. God help me help me help me please somebody help me ...

JUNE 15

I'm sick. I must be to keep having the images I have. I see myself taking my Henkel knife and cutting off my left hand, one sweet chop. Do I need medication? Should I be locked up in some institution? But I'm good 99% of the time. I haven't had an episode in over fifteen months. If I'd been locked up or on meds, I would have missed that amazing fifteen months of my life. Where does this monster come from? Why is it inside of me? It's me, a part of me anyway. Mostly I can keep the beast tamed, but I never know when it's going to rear its ugly head. That's why I don't think I can be a mother or hold down a real job. It used to take me out way more often and for longer. At least it's getting tamer.

Help obviously came. She sat with me and held my hand for a long time. I talked a bit and eventually calmed down. She put me to bed, and I eventually slept. It's a good thing she had me promise I wouldn't hurt myself. That kept me safe because I like to think that I honour my word, even in times of despair. The images still came at times but not as strong, the impulses even less. If only I had a gun, it would be so much easier.

I don't know what to do with myself today. I'm supposed to be hosting an event, a dance party, tonight. What a laugh! I guess I need to put my acting skills to use and put on a happy face. Who knows? That's ten hours away, anything could happen between now and then. Things could shift.

I have a session with Anjali in about twenty minutes. My friend kept telling me about remembering who I am, that I am love. What's the point of being love if there's no one to receive it, no one to share it with? Hardly anybody calls me, not even my family. My brother and sister never call. My parents rarely, if ever. Friends rarely, if ever. I don't even really have many friends. Theda and Monika. That's pretty much it. I blew my friendship with Zyla. Everyone else in my life is an acquaintance, co-worker, mentor, student or fan. All circumstantial relationships. Nobody makes the effort or shows the desire to really get to know me. I guess that's another reason why I'm writing this book—to feel known. To have an outlet, to be heard, to be seen. To feel like I exist. To validate my existence even? The only person who I think would be totally lost without me is my mom. Everyone else would be fine. They've got lots of other people and things going on in their lives. God, imagine what would happen if my mom died. I'd be totally fucked. I'm so weak, I can't handle loss well. When my grandma died, I locked myself up in my bedroom for days and wouldn't talk to or see anyone.

I had a good long session with Anjali. Two hours of working through stuff, my psyche. We ended with the process, "Why are you so alone?" I am loaded with ideas and beliefs about why I'm alone and not loveable: I'm fucked up, there's something wrong with me, I'm not good enough, I'm too much to handle, I'm a mess … and so on. It ended with a core belief, "Because my father didn't want me." He left when I was a child, would rarely visit. And when I did spend time with him on holidays, he was usually working and left me with other people. Then when we did start to connect and get to know each other, I constantly felt judged and criticised by him, and it seemed like whatever I did wasn't right or good enough. As a child this left a deep impression on me, of course, and him being the primary masculine role in my life … voila, men always leave me or won't seemingly love me for who I am. Even though I've worked on this issue a lot already and thought I'd resolved it, Anjali thinks that I may have resolved it logically, but that an emotional component hasn't been resolved. The wounded child is still hurting. She's offered me 2-hour sessions ongoing with no charge. She's an angel. It helps knowing someone cares about my emotional and mental well-being and happiness and is willing to help me.

It was fascinating. As I was telling Anjali the part about my dad, he called me. I have a pretty good relationship with my dad now. I think I've mentioned before that I've consciously worked really hard on it—we both have. But I guess it's the unconscious stuff that's still interfering with my life.

Also, interesting how it's Father's Day this weekend. I haven't done any work on my radio show and don't feel inspired to do it. We'll see. I was thinking that I might just put on a pre-recorded show. But then, there's my commitment to my sponsor, Hollyhock. We'll see. I just want to hole up in my bedroom and not see or talk to anyone. I guess the one good thing that's come out of all this is that I've been writing again. Good juicy drama for you, the reader. Got to keep it compelling, right?! ;-) Well, look at that, you got a wink and a smile out of me. Things are looking up.

June 16

Anjali and I are working at dismantling my mind. The mind frick, that is. The part that thinks that 'there's something wrong with me.' Thinking that there's something wrong with me is an idea that I have, that I'm quite convinced of actually. This idea is so imbedded in me that I think that it's real. I'm sure it's who I am. At times. Thankfully, not all the time. But I'm very good at convincing myself. I have lots of proof. I'm sure I could convince you of it, too. Let's see … I'm a middle-aged woman who has seasonal, on-call work; has had no success at any long-term relationships; has suicidal thoughts; has impulses for self-mutilation; has no major belongings or savings—in fact is in debt; has no major accomplishments; sleeps with a stuffed lion; gets upset when nobody calls or people don't come to my party; is emotionally unstable and immature; is lethargic and lazy and so on. Pretty convincing, right?!

That's one perspective of who I am. Obviously not a very loving or supportive one.

I had an insight while I was out for a walk. If I am coming from a place that 'there's something wrong with me,' of course I would need to find 'true love.' Finding true love would validate that 'I'm okay' and 'I'm loveable.' I'm not sure if that's completely my motivation for finding true love, but it could be. Definitely something to be aware of. I know I do need to strengthen my own belief in myself and cultivate self-love and acceptance.

I also had a moment when I paused to watch a red-headed wood-pecker, and I realized that I would be crazy to leave this place. This is a magical, beautiful paradise, and I should be grateful to be here, do everything in my power to stay, create a life here and trust that I will find someone who will want to co-create a life here with me. I would be miserable in Edmonton suburbia or even Victoria suburbia, for that matter. I think, I don't know. Does it matter where I am? I think it does. I need nature to nurture and inspire me. I can't make the mistake I made with past relationships. I need to learn from the past, get clear on what's important to me and to find someone who shares my passions, interests and values. Duncan said he did but obviously not enough to take any risks.

JUNE 17

I am so not in the zone right now. I was at a presenter evening at Hollyhock where people were talking about gratitude and faith and about being blessed. And they shared about how great life is. I could remember a time when I felt that way, but those feelings are so far from how I am feeling now—it's ridiculous. Instead, I feel full of dread, regret, remorse, loss, confusion, frustration, disappointment and letdown—and so on. I am stuck in a rut, a rut of my own misery and suffering, and I can't seem to get out. I guess it's just where I'm at and all I can do is accept it, be with it and, as everyone keeps telling me, trust and know that 'this too shall pass.'

I reread the first twenty pages of my book. I was in such a great place back then. I haven't kept any of the commitments to myself. I haven't been doing the things that bring me joy and that contribute to my well-being. Why do I keep giving up on myself?

The presenter evening I went to was about writing and perform-ing. I could have taken that workshop, but I didn't. Even though just four months ago, I was talking about how writing and performing were two things that I absolutely love and want to pursue. I keep losing myself, which feels shitty, but I ran into a friend today who talked about how there isn't really a 'self.' The 'self' is an illusion, and that's where I start to get all confused about reality again. What's real? What's true? What matters? If there is no self and life is meaningless, what's the point of it all? Why even bother? Especially if I'm not enjoying it. If I was enjoying 'the play,' then sure why not? But if I'm just suffering in it, why bother? It's all such a mind fuck. I guess I'll just keep working on dismantling the mind frick and see what happens. I have another session with Anjali tomorrow. I'll let you know how it goes.

JUNE 19

I'm stuck between a place of barely living and not knowing how to die. I feel like a shell of a person just going through the motions, empty, lost, numb. I've been fantasizing of different ways I could end my life, but I have no will or courage to do any of them. I started to write my will but got stuck at who to leave my harp to. My mind is so stubborn and won't loosen its grip on the idea that something's wrong with me; in fact, the idea just keeps getting stronger and, as I plot my own death, the proof stacks up against me.

Inspired by the movie *Seven Pounds*, I looked into donating my organs and such for the lives of others and thought there may be a way to donate my organs willingly and sacrifice my life for the benefit of others, but the law is that doctors must do everything in their power to keep you alive. I should be able to choose to die in a dignified way that contributes to the well-being of others, shouldn't I? So many lives are lost pointlessly, yet if we were given the option to give our lives so that others could live, wouldn't that be better? Ending suffering on so many levels and for so many people. How did death become such a terrible thing? Who decided life was preferable?

I sent in an application to become a UN volunteer. I decided that I'm too selfish and self-absorbed. As a lot of my suffering is caused by feelings of abandonment, my greatest gift could be giving love and care to those who have truly lost their parents. I need to do something bigger with my life, something that makes a greater impact and difference, something to get me out of my own misery. I realized that I can't be a mother or a wife anyway; I'm too unstable, too crazy, too self-absorbed. Why would I want to subject others to my misery? That would be selfish and irresponsible. I've been wanting a husband and children to fill the void, thinking that they would 'fix' me or make me into a better person. I am who I am—forty-one years. How can I expect to change? It's time I stopped trying to be something or someone I'm not, trying to portray someone that others will like and hopefully love.

Maybe it would be best that I go on medication. I don't know. I have another session with Anjali tomorrow but this baby's a tough nut to crack. Bedrock. It would take a miracle to turn my life around at this point. This book is a joke, too. Who's going to be interested in reading a crazy woman's ramblings with poor grammar and little imagination? This book was a 'fix,' too. False solutions—all of it. Time to wake up and face the reality of my life. Stop the visions of grandeur, the fantasies, the faery tales. My life is what it is, and I don't think I'm destined for anything that great.

JUNE 20–27

This was a very potent time, a lot happened that I wasn't able to capture in the moment so I'm going to do my best to capture it now. I remember that on the Wednesday I was at my friend Monika's hanging out in the backyard with her and her children, when our friend, Jen, came by and started talking about the Indigenous Leaders Gathering. Hearing about it sparked something in me. When I asked her when it was, she said it was that coming weekend. I instantly knew that I was meant to be there. I happened to have the next few days off and arranged to get another day off with ease. My dear friend and soul sister, Theda, and I had already made plans to get together anyway. When I called to see if she would be willing to go with me, she was instantly on board. The planning all came together quite smoothly.

We met up in Nanaimo and headed on our adventure together. The Gathering was in Lillooet. We had a fun and powerful road trip up the coast together. Our time together is always full and rich. I believe we did a dyad of some sort, but I can't remember what about. I do remember that just before we arrived in Whistler, I had a deep and profound revelation. I called Anjali and shared it with her on her voicemail. Later Anjali told me it was so clear and strong that she ended up saving that voicemail. I experienced a shift in consciousness and came to the realization that any attachment to the external would perpetuate suffering, so my project became deepening my connection within my Self, to that which never changes or goes away. The abiding Self. It seems so obvious and simple now but, at the time, I remember it creating such a sense of liberation and openness in me. Once again, my hardship was guiding me to Spirit and guiding me to connect on a deeper level to my own soul.

The Indigenous Leaders Gathering was profound. I experienced deep and powerful healing on many levels. I got to re-connect to a deep soul sister who I hadn't seen in a long time, and she was also recovering from a broken heart. There were leaders from all over the world: Nepal, Africa, China, North America and Peru. The woman leader from Africa spoke right to my heart

*about forgiveness and love. We Pow Wowed in the pouring rain with light-
ning and thunder for hours. I participated in an incredibly potent sweat lodge
with over thirty people in which I released and healed a lot in my heart and
psyche. I remember going up to the sweat leaders at the end of the sweat and
telling them I had a revelation about leadership—that it needs to change on
a large scale. I asked them how that can happen and they told me, "It starts
with you, in how you are and the things that you do, the way you interact
with people, the example you set." Of course. It always starts with us. With
me. I'm doing my best. That's all any of us can do. Do our best. When we
falter, try again. Learn from our mistakes and move on. Over and over again
as long as it takes. Never give up, my friend. It starts with us ...*

JUNE 28

I don't know how to make peace with life. I don't get it. I don't understand it. I'm not enjoying it. My grandpa's in a coma, and he's not likely to come out. He was driving just last week, dancing a little while before that. I have some regrets. Not going to visit him last time I was in Alberta, not spending last Christmas with him at my mom's, not going to his ninetieth birthday party. I'll never get another chance to play a game with him or dance with him. What can I do? I could focus on the positive. I did see him at my mom's last fall and we played a lot of games together. I talked to him on the phone frequently. I'll miss his funny sounds and the way he used to call me BJ. I don't even know why he did. *My grandpa passed away that evening. This was my tribute to him:*

Dad, Poppa, Grandpa as described by some as witty, kind, caring, playful, hardworking and as a wonderful teacher. There was a quiet love about him.

A free spirit who loved to dance, build things, play cards and tricks. Poppa made great funny sounds and laughed lots.

I will treasure all the games, the laughs and the fun times had with him.

We love you, miss you, God Bless & Rest In Peace.

June 29

Be at least as interested in what goes on inside you as what happens outside. If you get the inside right, the outside will fall into place.
~ Eckhart Tolle

Wow, it's a fascinating journey, this getting to know one's self. A definite unending unfolding mystery. I feel like I might be actually 'growing up' or maybe it would be more apt to say, 'waking up.' I sense that life is maturing me in a way, forcing me to come into my own, so to speak. Yeah, big wake up calls. Heartbreak, death, loss, hardship. It makes me think of my 'destiny card' and the way it told me that I am destined to keep experiencing hardship to force me closer to Spirit. That so rings true. I've started to study the Kabbalah. Well, I've been called to explore it, and I happened to have a book that my second mom, Marilyn, gave me quite a while ago called, *Ecstatic Kabbalah* by Rabbi David A. Cooper. It even has meditations in it and an accompanying CD. I've been doing twenty to thirty minutes of practice a day as it recommends. Plus I've been meditating at least twenty-four minutes a day of mindful witness practice plus more than thirty minutes of Yoga Nidra every morning plus a commitment to get on my mat at least once a day even if just for ten or thirty minutes. I feel I'm going deeper into pratyahara, exploring this connection to Source within.

PRATYAHARA

Pratyahara is the fifth limb of yoga, and it is concerned with taking us from the outside to the inside by withdrawing the senses, so that the yogi, like an inner-naut, can travel within and find the Self.[21]

Wow, I get so easily distracted. I have my email open, and I saw the subject of an email that said, "Stop Bill C38." So I had to look at it, and it had a link to a petition so I went there, and then I had to post it to Facebook so I went there, and then I started reading people's posts and then I started chatting with my Auntie Brenda about Poppa.

I was talking to a couple this evening at Hollyhock about ADHD as they had just taken a workshop with Gabor Mate. Gabor claims to have it and has written a book on it. I mentioned that I thought I had a bit of it, and I guess the previous paragraph is the proof. I can't seem to stay focussed on any one thing for very long, but I love what they shared about what he said about it, that it enables him to do many different things.

Okay, enough said. It's getting late, gotta go to bed. I'll have a lot of time to write in the next five days. I'm doing a writing workshop, Writing Sesshin with Ruth Ozeki. *Remember when I called in a woman mentor to teach me about writing? Voila! Things that make you go hmmm ...*

JUNE 30

I see my mind getting all kinds of lofty ideas and hopes as it tends to do, imagining that I'll complete my book during this workshop. Five days of meditating and writing! For sure! And yet the wiser part of me is beginning to understand that life is not about the goals and the outcome, life is about accepting where I'm at, being present and enjoying the moment, the journey. And yet, as I write that, I question that too. It's probably a combination of both, of course.

I'm sitting in the Hollyhock garden surrounded by the buzz of busy bees as they gather pollen from the multitude of flowers that are in full glorious bloom. Reds, oranges, blues, purples, magentas, pinks—colours exploding everywhere. I really like what Ruth shared yesterday; she said that she learned from one of her teachers: "It's important to accept the writer that I am, no matter how different I wish myself to be. I am the writer that I am." That's both liberating and empowering. We each have a story to tell through a unique voice, a unique perspective. I find it fascinating that at times I feel I have so much to share. I get overtaken with an urgency to have you know my entire world, my whole experience of life and, other times, I think, "How futile, how naïve and childish. Who would want to know about me?" I guess I just have to trust that part of me that feels compelled to share.

I was thinking during my bike ride to Hollyhock earlier that even though I don't know how, I sense that my writing is intended to be of benefit to someone. Especially with my willingness and ability to write about my darkest experiences. Perhaps someone reading it will be touched in a way that lets them know they are not alone or they aren't the only one who struggles. And reading my story will be that ray of hope or light that gets them through the challenges or darkness. I don't know. I am curious what writing is about, especially when some say we need to let go of our stories and of our past to be more present in the moment. Perhaps the telling of our stories is a way of letting them go even though, in some way, it seems to solidify them. I guess the key is to not allow our stories to limit us and to recognize that we are not bound by them. Yes, they do mold and form us in some way, but we are not just our stories—we are so much more.

I get these moments in which I feel overwhelmed by my own thoughts and consciousness and think that there's too much to process or capture into words. Words don't do my experience or awareness any justice. I guess that's another reason why I don't talk very much. Often times in sharing circles, when asked to express a word or a phrase that captures our experience, instead of words, sound and movement are what come out. And yet I'm choosing a path of writing and not dancing?! Sometimes I don't understand myself. Maybe that's the reason why I'm embarking on this path of writing, so I can explore this mode of expression to better understand myself. I can express myself freely and easily through sound and movement, and now it's time to hone my skill of communication through words. God knows I definitely struggle with that. Oh yeah, I decided to not worry about what I share with you in this book because of the power of editing. I was starting to get concerned about the 'appropriateness' and 'relevancy' and so on bullshit of what I should and how I should be sharing/writing. I decided to let all that go; I can decide in the editing process. That's why there's such a thing as editing. That takes some pressure off. I don't have to 'get it right.'

It is challenging to know or decide about what to share. There's so much going on. I'll pause to breathe, feel into my body and see what emerges. Recalling the title and intention of this book, *From My Heart To Yours* ...I breathe into my heart while also feeling outward into yours and see what comes.

Something about Buddha is emerging. I recall the dharma talk I went to way back in April. And I remember being struck about Buddha's big realizations and wake-up call. His experience of samvega. He was struck by illness, aging and death and realized that they were all inevitable. I think part of me has been in this deluded state that I could somehow avoid or transcend those experiences, and this spring has been about me waking up to the impending reality of illness, aging and death. It's maturing me in some way, deepening me, pulling me out of my bubble of denial. Even though it's been painful, it feels like a good thing. Like I'm getting a missing piece of the puzzle of life. I still have so many questions, uncertainties and misunderstandings about life, existence and myself.

Oh, I did have a realization earlier how I am such a mystery who is continually unfolding and actually how exciting that is. Life can be so beautiful when I surrender to that 'not knowing.' It's fascinating how life is this continual cycle of forgetting and remembering, getting lost and being found, resistance and acceptance, the holding on and the letting go. The piece I keep getting reminded of, during it all, is to keep my heart open. Don't let anything shut me down or close me off. And luckily so far, that's the one thing I seem to be able to keep coming back to. Is it really all about love? Is love really all there is? If so, what exactly is it? There are so many misconceptions and ideas of what love is and isn't. I guess that's part of the journey of life: exploring and discovering the different ways to experience and express love, being and not being love or, at least, seeming to not be love. But if love is all there is, then it's all love, even when it seems it might not be, right? I make myself giggle when I go into these mind fricks. It is wild how I can go from being totally 'in love' with myself and my life to being totally 'out of love' in the span of weeks, days or even hours.

Such a vast array of experiences to be had in this human form. I still don't know what it's all about—this human experience, that is. The jury's still out on that one, and perhaps I'll never know. And maybe that's the point—coming back to the not knowing thing again. A-ha, there's the rub. That truly is where the magic is, in the willingness to not know ... to be willing to sit and move through the mystery. That place of childlike wonder and curiosity. Being open to all possibilities and willing to be surprised. I love surprises, I love being in that place of wonder and possibility. Then why this incessant drive 'to know'?! Habit, I guess. Supposedly it's one of the most prevalent universal addictions. The need to know.

FOUR UNIVERSAL ADDICTIONS

In *The Four-Fold Way*, anthropologist Angeles Arrien identifies four basic human addictions. These are "life-negating" patterns that underlie all addictions, whether to drugs, food, work, sex, etc. These four basic addictions are:

1) The addiction to intensity. This shows up when love is lacking.

2) The addiction to perfection. This appears when true excellence is misunderstood and true power is unrealized.

3) The addiction to knowledge. This is the opposite of wisdom.

4) The addiction to focusing on what's not working rather than what is working. What's missing here is seeing the big picture.

It's fascinating to be in this place where I feel a big shift is coming, even needed. And yet, at the same time, that knowing that I need to be at peace with and to accept where I'm at. That paradoxical pull once again. The pull to be and the pull to evolve. I am recalling a moment I had during an Enlightenment/ Illumination Intensive in which I had a visceral and energetic experience of birthing myself anew in each moment. Each moment an opportunity to be reborn, a letting go of the old and an embracing of the new. Each breath, a new possibility. I feel myself coming more alive as I write about this, as I remember, as I let go, as I breathe myself more and more into being, into this present moment.

I pause to take in the beauty of my surroundings, the vivid colours, the fluttering of butterfly wings, the songs of the birds, the expansiveness of the sky, the caress of the breeze, the fresh scent of ocean air. My legs are falling asleep, my butt hurts and I have to pee, from the profound to the profane in one fell swoop. That's life, isn't it?!

If I use the metaphor of garden for my life, this is what I see. I just walked around the Hollyhock garden for the last 15 minutes taking in the incredible beauty and perfection of decades of ongoing loving attention and energy by master gardeners. I recall my own garden, over run with weeds, stunted growth, struggling plants, half-eaten leaves and non-germinating seeds. I can be discouraged and disheartened by seeing how pathetic and sorry my garden is compared to Hollyhock's, or I can be inspired and motivated by seeing the potential of what's possible with ongoing care and attention. There's so much potential within each of us for anything really. It's what and where we choose to focus our energy. Even though I have zero experience as a mother, it doesn't mean that I don't have the potential to be a great one. What I really mean to say is that I don't have to know something in order to do it or be it. I can learn and grow into anything I choose—well, almost anything. Not sure if I could grow into an Olympic athlete at this point in my life but I did hear about someone who decided to become a doctor in his forties. How much of our life is determined by choice and how much by circumstance and fate? This is the ongoing question for me. Does it really matter? I guess all I can do is keep making choices when given the opportunity and accept the things that I don't choose when they come. That makes me think of the serenity prayer:

God grant me the serenity
to accept the things I cannot change;
courage to change the things I can;
and wisdom to know the difference.

Got distracted by the net and started surfing Facebook. Sometimes it's good to get distracted and gain a new perspective. This is what I found:

There are two basic motivating forces: fear and love.
When we are afraid, we pull back from life. When we are
in love, we open to all that life has to offer with passion,
excitement, and acceptance. We need to learn to love
ourselves first, in all our glory and our imperfections. If we
cannot love ourselves, we cannot fully open to our ability
to love others or our potential to create. Evolution and all
hopes for a better world rest in the fearlessness and
open-hearted vision of people who embrace life.
~ John Lennon

I keep being drawn back to the issue of self-love. As if it would solve all of life's problems. Is it truly possible to completely love one's self? When I recall the times that I felt in love with myself, those times of complete acceptance and enjoyment of who I am and my life as it is, life was amazing. I was in the zone, in the flow. Life and relationships flowed with grace, ease, sweetness and harmony. I don't have to have it all figured out. It's a life-long project, a journey, an adventure of exploration, discovery, co-creation, accepting, letting go. All of it to be marvelled at and enjoyed to the best of one's ability. The question arose: "What's my plight in all this?" I looked up the definition of 'plight' in the Free Dictionary online: "A situation, especially a bad or unfortunate one." But then I looked further and this is what I found:

1. To promise or bind by a solemn pledge, especially to betroth.

2. To give or pledge (one's word or oath, for example).

n. A solemn pledge, as of faith.

One's word. Faith. All deep and profound inquiries. I'm continually astounded by how infrequently people honour their word these days. I guess I should look at myself. I could definitely tighten up in that area. Faith is something I have an ongoing struggle with. I came to the conclusion during one of my sessions with Anjali that with 'faith,' nothing would phase me. It would all be okay, and I would be okay with anything and everything. Faith seems to be the anchor to calm, peace, acceptance and to grace. If only I could believe in myself more, trust in the natural unfolding of life. It's coming. Again, an ongoing project. The project of life. "Terrible fun," as Anjali puts it. Terrible fun, indeed! *She has since changed it to 'awful fun' ... 'awe-full fun,' which I like even better!*

JULY 1

The fabric of life—each aspect an integral thread in the weave of existence. So is the same of me, each aspect of my being is an essential and necessary piece in the mosaic that I am. The unique manifestation, creation, expression of me. These are the thoughts and realizations that came to me as I sat and walked on the beach. Taking it all in: the air, the sky, the clouds, the mountains, the trees, the ocean, the birds, insects, seaweed, fish, sun. A deep appreciation.

I woke up tired this morning and wondered how much was due to habit and how much was real. The question, "How much is my choice?" Oh, I'm remembering what came to me as I was balancing on the rocks on the beach and lamenting the loss of the fun and playful side of me. It's still here, it's in me. I get to choose when she comes out. I haven't lost her. She's in me as are all aspects of being. Different strokes for different folks. Different situations, people and influences will evoke different aspects of my being, if I choose. It's up to me as to how much I let myself be influenced by the external. I think. I'm not totally sure.

I think I'm trying too hard. Nothing wants to come. I don't feel like I have anything to say. I feel I need to come back to that place of writing just for the sake of writing. I stare up at the clouds hoping for some inspiration. I close my eyes and take a few deep breaths: my jaw loosens, I yawn, I let out a sigh. I sink into myself, into my current experience. A settling, a deepening while also expanding my awareness to include my surroundings. My senses alert and at the ready—I'm wanting so desperately to sound brilliant, profound and wise. I smile and snicker to myself: amused or bemused—I'm not sure which, maybe both—by my predictability. That sweet tender part of me that wants so badly to be liked, to be heard, to be understood. I am learning to be gentler with her, to give her space and a voice. A softening, a nodding of my head in that sweet knowing that this is good—because it is, it simply is. I wish I could be this kind and gentle and loving to myself all the time. Imagine how different life would be. Imagine the energy I would have available. Imagine the freedom. I tasted that this afternoon, when I went for that walk on the beach, then swam naked in the ocean, danced and did Qi Gong on the sand. When I know that feeling of freedom and joy is possible, why don't I allow myself to feel it more often? So often bound by fear, consideration, concern, self-consciousness, judgment, appropriateness. Donna Martin's words come to mind, "Consciousness loves contrast."

What am I here for? What's my unique offering? Blech ... that broken record. Boggling how it keeps resurfacing even after I've answered those questions, what seems like, a hundred thousand times.

I have been meaning to share a profound realization I had mid-April, in connection to the tarot reading I had and have shared with you. I was on the ferry from Nanaimo to Horseshoe Bay; the sun was setting and, as I stood there on the outside deck and looked out at the brilliant crimson sky, I 'got it.' I got what my unique expression/gift is to the world. It's me! Simply and wonderfully me. As long as I continue to share and express myself authentically from my heart, I am the gift. That is my unique offering and it/I will take many different forms depending on the day, time, place, influences, surroundings, people, and so on. The form doesn't matter. I don't have to 'figure out' what my unique offering is as it is bound to continually change over and over. The constant, the essence, is me. I'm not sure if I'm capturing it and expressing it fully, but you probably get the gist. It was an exquisite moment when I got it. I felt so present, so alive, so free and ... and what? I can't quite describe it in words. Almost like validated, I guess. I was moved to tears, it was a homecoming. Perhaps a mini satori even. Such a sweet and precious moment. One I need to keep remembering.

A deer just came over the ridge, walking towards me, ears and tail flickering, nose sniffing. She's sussing me out, and I guess she's decided I'm harmless. She's grazing on the lush grass of the lawn beside me, under the apple tree. An eagle screeches from his perch on the tree top just to the other side of me; another calls in response as it soars overhead. I feel my heart. Three eagles now, the deer grazing even closer. I sit in awe, a feeling of bewilderment, as if nature has responded to my moment of awakening. A feeling of expansion in my heart, a smile, a knowing that all is good, all is as it should be. A sigh of relief. That includes me. Cultivate and build the trust in myself—that's all that's required. Everything else I need is here, in me and around me. It always comes back to that, trust and faith. The deer is scratching its ear with its hind leg—so adorable, so reassuring how comfortable and safe she feels. She nibbles at her back. Such an honour. I'm given this honour a lot, the trust of others. Now it's time to give it to myself.

July 2

Life affirming, reclaiming, liberating, empowering. Writing! I'm not the only one who thinks I'm crazy, I mean who 'thinks that they're crazy.' It's actually a common trait amongst writers. I also feel that I've finally found a calling in which my incessant questioning is an attribute. I think I may have found 'my tribe.' One of them anyway. It feels good. I feel more whole and complete.

JULY 3

A writing exercise from the workshop, to write about oneself in third person:

She found cover just in the nick of time, the hand-painted green sign read 'Kids Space.' Posted above a driftwood arched entrance that she had to duck to get through. There was a miniature picnic table in the corner. The walls, made of graying knotted wood came to her hip, a half wall, the upper half left open to look out at the beautiful surrounding scenery. Ocean, trees, rocks, sky, clouds, sailboats, floating islands, passing deer, soaring eagles. She set her things down on the table, took out her laptop, sat at the miniature table, her knees poking out to the sides, and began to write. She paused to listen to the sound of the raindrops hitting the roof. A heron hollers nearby. She looks out, her favourite! Sun showers! "There must be a rainbow somewhere!" she thinks excitedly. She looks expectantly all around, greens of trees and grass, grey and blue of ocean and sky, white of daisies and clouds, browns of driftwood, seaweed and rocks, yellow of dandelions dot the lawn, but no arc of colour to be seen.

The press of possibility suffocated her making it impossible to simply enjoy herself. The voice of judgment stifling any sense of joy. "You're so contained," and "If you were more free you'd be barefoot and naked, running and dancing in the sand ..."

Rain on face, wind in hair, the flap of her light cotton sweater like wings, the crunch of sand, shell and rock beneath her feet. The bubbling of clams bring back memories of the snap, crackle, pop of Rice Krispies just after milk is added.

My deep thought for the day: "Writing is like metta, sending out thoughts to others, for yours and their benefit."

July 5

"I am the writer that I am." The words of her writing guru played over and over in her head like a mantra combating the feelings of inadequacy and doubt.

I feel like I'm living a half-life, and I have no profound reasons such as accidently killing someone to justify this pathetic existence. (I make reference to Darin Straus' life and book, *Half a Life*). The word 'pathetic' seems too drastic, but I couldn't think of the right one so it will do for now. It feels strange to be in this in-between place, this place where, on one hand, I know I have a pretty good, if not great life, and know that I am blessed to be where I am, doing what I'm doing. I'm good at what I do; in fact, I'm really fucking good. I touch people in profound and meaningful ways. I live in paradise. I have a lot of free time to do what I want. And yet, I feel such lethargy and blahness, and I'm getting sick and tired of hearing myself complain. What the fuck!? How do I break out of this slump?

I started a parasite cleanse today. That means no sweets for at least a month, maybe longer. And, of course, I'm craving chocolate like crazy!! I have so much criticism running through my head, I'm so not loving myself right now. I feel scattered and unfocussed, thinking I need to be more productive and all I want to do is distract myself with a movie. What's the better thing to do? Push on and try to force myself to do something? Or give in to what I'm feeling and just watch the damn movie? Why do I make such a big fucking deal out of it? I need to have more fun. I'm too uptight these days. Too serious. Yep, I need to lighten up. Perhaps that means watching a comedy! ;-) I think I'll write for a little while longer and then reward myself with a movie. There! Compromise—a beautiful thing. The middle way, yes and yes! That feels better. Honouring both sides, both pulls.

I'm trying to avoid the feelings of loneliness that keep trying to seep in. I've decided to give up on my faery tale notion of true love and to let the whole attachment to finding a partner and having a family go. On some level, I feel healthier, less idealistic and naïve. On the other hand, I feel kind of sad that I've lost that innocent notion of love. I'm still open to the possibility, but I need to let go of the attachment and the neediness. I'm watching two hummingbirds zip around outside, they're such a delight to watch. So full of life. I've lost my mojo, and I need to get it back. My joie de vivre! Where is it? Where did it go? How do I get it back?

I've been wondering if I should rewrite my book as fiction. It may be safer and more interesting that way. Supposedly novels sell much better than non-fiction. It could be fun to retell my story with the creative license to embellish. But then, it would lose that raw realness that I was going for. Or maybe not. I've never tried writing fiction. It could open up a whole new world. I could let my imagination run wild, I could live out all my fantasies. Maybe that's what I've been needing. Instead of trying to force this world to fit my idea of how it should be, I can actually create new worlds, people and situations—exactly as I want them. Wow! What a power. Writing fiction is like playing God! How fascinating. How enticing!! ;-) Now that got me a little juiced. I actually feel a little bit of excitement and energy in my solar plexus and heart. Hmmm … what might be cool is to blend the two, fiction and nonfiction, and see what comes from that. Kind of like those cartoon and real people movies, such as *Waking Life*.

I feel like something's broken inside of me. Something that doesn't allow me to fully connect with and enjoy my own experience of life. Or even life itself. I have all this awareness of the good in my life, but I can't seem to really connect with it. It feels separate. I feel separate. Despite all the work, all the training, all the meditation, therapy, yoga, sacred journeys, none of it seems to be able to repair this disconnect. How do other people cope? What do other people do with their limiting beliefs and shitty attitudes? I think I need to get out in nature more. Or meditate more or both. There's the constant 'more' factor. Never enough, too much, more of this more of that. Less … argh!!!! I feel so frustrated and irritated right now. Yes, definitely time to go meditate.

July 7

Self-acceptance, self-love ... such a foreign concept. Is it truly possible? If so how? Am I destined to be alone until this elusive promise of salvation? So packed full of judgments, criticisms. So bound by my own suffocating ideas of who I am and who I think I should be. Trapped behind the walls of my own misery and sense of separation. Will these walls ever come down? They seem to be made by some unknown and equally impenetrable material. The mass/ bedrock of my mind. Fortified by the pounding of my thoughts, decade after decade.

July 8

Stephen Cope seems to be writing right to/for me. Crazy how I know this stuff, too, but he puts it in a way that makes so much sense. Breathe, Relax, Feel, Watch, Allow (BRFWA). So simple, yet so powerful. I have to stop denying my experience and trying to change it. I realized today that I'm still grieving and that I need to give myself space for that. I can't expect to be all chipper, bright and cheery. It's totally understandable that I'm feeling a bit glum. It's okay. I feel myself soften a little at that notion, and a spontaneous big breath enters my body. Practise practise practise.

I need to stop abandoning myself. My avoidance of my yoga practice is a perpetuation of this dishonouring. I think from a childish place of wanting to be saved—the unwillingness to accept that I was abandoned. I need to accept that, grieve it and commit to being there for myself.

I just had a major shift in the bath. I practised the BRFWA and caught myself every time my thoughts or attention would wander away. So much became clear, my whole pattern … it goes like this …

My cycle:

I start opening up to someone or a group or a community and am excited to share and connect. At some point, I hit a deep imbedded wall of insecurity and get self-conscious and self-critical. I start to pull back. Feelings of shame and guilt build up and fortify the wall of separation. I start to feel more and more disconnected and, with the disconnection, I have feelings of loneliness and despair. Not wanting to burden others with these darker more negative feelings, I withdraw even more. My interactions and connections with others become less and less frequent and more and more fake and forced. I start feeling stuck and hopeless and don't know how to bridge the gap or break out of my fortress of isolation. Life starts to become lifeless and meaningless without connection, laden with the weight

From My
Heart
To Yours

of so much self-loathing. I lose touch with what's real, with life itself. It takes a huge amount of effort to reach out and ask for help, to establish any kind of contact. Eventually I re-emerge with a lot of help from friends, mentors and family reminding me of who I am and my ability to connect.

Hummingbirds abound.

July 10

Every time I go to write, I get swept by this wave of fatigue and just want to go have a nap instead. So I'm writing anyway. Just to break through that block of resistance. I've been feeling stuck again lately. Unsure of what to write about. Unsure of how to write. I've been feeling tired a lot lately, so yesterday I did an exercise where I sat down and opened up a dialogue with my body and wrote down some questions: Okay, body, what are you trying to tell me? What are you needing and wanting from me? I'm here to listen and I will not abandon you anymore. And this is what it said in response: "I need more rest. Stillness, more conscious breathing. Conscious letting-go time. Surrender Yoga. Sleep. Fresh foods. Less sugar. More water. Gentleness, kindness, acceptance. Loving touch. Long walks in the trees. Deeper connections. Slow down. Be present. Eat slower and more consciously. Softer, smoother. Laughter, play, fun. Less worry and concern. Yes, more stillness, more listening. Gentle rocking, gentle dancing, swaying. Floating in the water. More space to feel. Acceptance. More alone time. Me dates. Self-exploratory pleasuring."

July 16

What if everything you did was an act of love for yourself or someone else? What would life be like? What if everyone lived that way? What kind of world would we be living in? If love is all there is, then from one perspective, it's already so, but that's definitely hard to believe.

It's been an amazing week. I've been so present to how incredible my life is and how blessed I am. I live in paradise. I get paid to love others or guide them to love themselves. I get to swim naked in the ocean at my workplace. I get to see deer and fawns graze outside my studio window. I get to meet amazing people from all over the world. I get to drink clean water right out of my tap; I get to breathe clean air. Beauty abounds and surrounds me everywhere I look. I have a good balance of work and free time. I get to swim, dance, play music, write and do yoga. Yep, it's a rough life but somebody's gotta live it! ;-) I guess this is the reward for all of the suffering I went through. It probably makes me appreciate my blessings all the more. I was thinking earlier while I was at the beach, "What makes a good piece of writing? The fact that someone is willing to reveal and express themselves authentically and share that with others?" Can it be that simple? Is that simple? Not so much. But I know there is 'bad' writing out there. Or maybe there isn't—maybe it just depends on who's reading it. Like 'one man's junk is another man's treasure,' one piece of writing may be shit to one person, but another may love it. I think it's about trusting and owning that I have a voice, that I have something in me to say and share and that someone—hopefully many someones—will enjoy hearing it. Then the question arises, "Does it matter?" Should it matter? Why does it matter? Can I just write for writing sake? This need to be heard, seen, known, understood. Is it okay? Is it natural? Healthy? I guess it's there, so it's gotta be okay on some level. Especially if I come back to loving myself as I am. Sure there's always room for improvement and, perhaps someday, those needs will shift, morph and change as all things do. But right now, that's just the way it is. So I write because I enjoy it and because I want you to read it. And so it is.

August 13

It's been a long time since my last entry (my confession). I had this realization that I've done to you what Duncan has done to me—acted as if you don't exist and withdrawn all of my attention, my love. And in abandoning you, I've abandoned myself. This book is like—no, it IS a relationship. It needs ongoing love, attention, care, respect and commitment.

It's wild how much certain things teach me about myself and my ability to relate to others. I've felt quite withdrawn as of late. Not completely but to a degree. Almost like an animal nursing its wounds. Still a little skittish, jittery, wary, tentative, afraid. I've been struggling with my tendency to focus on what's wrong. Both with me and with my life. Even though I focus on gratitude every day and all the incredible blessings in my life, I still get consumed with what's missing, what's not quite right. Even though every day and through-out the day, I focus on Loving Presence, compassionate awareness, acceptance, gratitude … it's so hard to break out of that habit of seeing what's wrong. Fascinating. Yes, life certainly is fascinating. Well, there's a lot more to say but it's late, and I just wanted to get some-thing down, to acknowledge where I'm at and to recommit to this relationship, to this unfolding. And see where it takes us. Round and round it goes, where it stops nobody knows … ;-)

August 14

Another beautiful day in paradise. I had really lovely sessions today, especially my first one. I believe we really accessed a sweet space of grace. It was quite lovely. During the session, I became aware of how my intention/practice is to be totally present with her in a space of loving acceptance, compassion and care. In doing that, I realized that the reason I struggle with that so much is because I don't give that to myself. If I want to shift my relationship with my work to one of more ease, grace and love, I need to shift my relationship with myself. I need to be more loving, accepting and compassionate with myself and my situation. Stop looking for or focussing on what's wrong, what's lacking, what needs to change, and so on. It's fascinating how difficult that is. How I'm so locked into that energy of criticalness, judgment, evaluation, assessment, and so forth.

I create a lot of unnecessary suffering when I get into that space of focussing on what's wrong. I just sent a message to Donna Martin about it, to see what advice she may have to help me and to perhaps start having ongoing sessions with her to work on it. It's at the core of my unhappiness and suffering—I am clear on that. Probably the only thing that I am clear on these days. Although I did get clear that I want to make my life about mastering Loving Presence, acceptance and compassion. That, until I do, nothing else really matters. During my session today, I realized how right they are when they say it's not 'what' you do, it's 'how' you do it that matters. So what's the point in getting any more training or switching to any other 'career' until I can be fully present in that space of loving acceptance and compassion in the work that I presently do? The reason I probably am not in a loving relationship is due to the fact that I don't love and accept myself as I am. If I don't, how can I expect somebody else to. Although it would be nice. ;-) See even that is me setting up a standard for myself: I must attain total self-love and acceptance before somebody else will love me. It's incessant. I do truly wonder if it's possible. Will I ever truly love and accept myself?

AUGUST 16

I was sitting out by the fire and felt a need to write. So here I am. There's been so much happening, moving through me. It's so hard to keep up. I had some moments of pure and utter joy today. I was swimming in the ocean, and I just spontaneously started laughing with joy. Pure, sweet, beautiful joy. The pure joy of being alive. Living in paradise. Ocean, mountains, heron nearby, sun, sand. I had the most amazing dance on the beach; it's become my favourite place to dance. I guess it's been that for a while, but I just forgot. I use to go every morning when I lived in Roberts Creek way back in 1999. Life is truly amazing when I am present to it. In it fully. Living it. It's when I begin to worry about what's going to happen in the future that I get concerned and suffer.

I am curious about what goes on in my body. I experience a lot of sensation that I would label as pain, and I'm not sure what to do about it. I can just feel it, be present and try my best to still have a good time, but it does take my attention. I was thinking today that I must hold some sort of belief system about needing to suffer for the benefit of others. It doesn't have to be that way. It's wild how in some sessions, I can come out feeling totally energized and good and, other times, I feel wiped, achy and drained. I have had some amazing sessions lately. I was able to be so present and hold a beautiful space of love, compassion and curiosity. That's when grace shows up; it is felt by both of us. I remembered that it's not what I do that matters but how I do it. Until I master being present, loving and compassionate with my life as it is, what's the point of taking on anything else? It's all a distraction and made-up goals to feel like I'm making progress or 'doing something' with my life. I want my life to be about Loving Presence, compassion, wonder, joy and acceptance.

I've been thinking that perhaps one of the reasons I can't seem to apply much or any discipline to my life is because the Divine

Intelligence is directing me to a more integrated lifestyle in which things aren't so delineated and separate. So instead of "I do yoga at this time," and "I meditate at this time," and "I do this practice at this time"—it all becomes a part of my everyday existence. For example, I was practicing presence, conscious breathing and gratitude while picking blueberries. I don't want to just be present, open and compassionate during my yoga practice; it's how I choose to live my life, every moment of every day.

I've been obsessed with eating lately, for quite a while actually. I can't seem to stop, even when I'm full or have just eaten a beautiful meal. As soon as I'm done, I think about what I can eat next. It's like I'm needing to fill myself. I'm not sure why. To stuff emotions? To feel full? To distract myself? For the pure sensuality of it, the taste, the texture? I'm not sure. I just want to keep eating. Sweet, salty, crunchy, silky, hot, cold, fresh, cooked, all over the place. I just want to keep stuffing myself.

I feel like I'm hiding out. I'm holding back. Not fully expressing, sharing nor living my true and full self. I'm not sure why. I'm aware of some self-consciousness, still some concern about what others think. It's amazing to experience those fleeting moments of freedom, raw and true being and expressing. So free, so fun, so alive. Why don't I live that way all the time? Why still so much concern about what others think? Oh, to be the full and true wild woman that I am. Eventually, little by little, like the ongoing unfolding of the lotus flower.

I am living a dream life. My dream life. I live in paradise. Clean air, clean water, ocean, lakes, forest, mountains, waterfalls, organic gardening, sustainable living, artists, musicians, creatives of all types, spiritual community, yoga, healing, celebration. It's my dream life and I'm living it. Damn, I really have to acknowledge that. I think sometimes I downplay it or don't really own it due to the guilt I feel because so many people are unhappy and not living their dream life. I think a part of me wonders if and how I deserve it. So I make shit up to create the illusion of suffering so I don't feel so guilty. But if I get really present to my life, it's fucking amazing!! Fantasy quality. Shit to write about. So here I am, finally getting back on track. It's amazing the stints of self-doubt, fear and crap I can get caught in. Trust. Gotta trust. Gotta remember the essence of what life is all about. Breathe easy, smile, remember. It's all good.

AUGUST 23

I am still concerned with receiving outside validation and approval. I'm still looking to be singled out as special. That little girl hoping to be discovered and made into a movie star. Spotted from across a crowded room and told "I'm the one" "I've captured his heart." Envy, envy of those who have found that, who have had 'special' encounters with 'special' people, which makes them 'special.'

I just re-watched *Eat, Pray, Love*. Argh, that stupid comparison thing. So deadly. Plus the guest staying with me has such incredible tales of adventure and a fully lived 'special' life. Why do I see myself in such poor light? So insignificant and unimportant? Why am I not enough? I feel stuck in some deep-seated pattern of self-loathing and self-deprecation. Feeling insufficient, broken, lost, simple. Simple is good though. But there's still that part of me that thinks I should be more, different, better.

While I was lying in the hammock today being present to the pain in my body, I had the thought that maybe I need to start getting curious about this pain that I live with because it's not going away and to see what it's trying to teach me. I also had the thought that if I was able to shift my eating habits and simply be able to eat with full presence—slowly and consciously—that my whole experience of life would change. It's amazing how difficult that seemingly simple task is. There are two very simple yet big projects to add to my practice. The others being to cultivate Loving Presence, compassionate awareness and gratitude. All very noble causes and yet, for my ambitious mind, not enough.

Where do I make money? How do I make a living? When do I make something of myself and my life? Ha! Funny stuff. I still have some hopes for this book. It's the only thing I have going for me right now so ... yep. It's amazing how I can see so many possible directions I can go, but I don't know how any of them will result in any type of 'fortune' or way of even simply supporting myself. And the frustrating thing is that I'm still obsessing about that. Why can't I just trust? Why am I still so caught up in that paradigm of 'making a living'? It's so not what I've ever been about nor want to be about, and yet it's always there lurking in the background. I guess it's that I do want to have more choices and freedom. I feel trapped in my lack of financial freedom. I also don't want to be a burden on anyone—family nor potential partner. I want to prove to myself that I can be self-sufficient. I would like to master the material/money realm so that I don't feel a victim to it anymore. I don't know why I struggle with it so much. I really do feel like I have some huge energetic or psychic block around money and self-sufficiency. It's quite fascinating really. I wonder where it comes from, what it's about and what I'm meant to learn from it.

I wish I trusted myself more. I believe that's a big missing piece—trusting and believing in myself. Confidence. I know that I have a lot to offer others and the world, and yet I hold a lot back due to lack of confidence. Then I come to the question, "Is my practice to accept where I am at or to work on building confidence?" Probably both. Or one comes with the other. Trust, trust the natural unfolding of life, of my being. And then the ongoing conundrum of how much do I surrender versus how much do I will into being? What's the difference? How do I know when to do which? Or which is which? Or does it matter? I love one of the quotes from the movie, *Eat, Pray, Love*: "God is inside of me as I am." But I don't know who that is. I have so many possibilities of expression. I don't know what my unique gifts are. And then I have those moments in which I get that I don't need to know. In fact, it's better if I don't, and I just trust and allow the natural unfolding of the mystery of who I am. Allow myself and others to be pleasantly surprised moment by moment. Such an incessant need to know. Oh, this crazy mind of mine. This crazy life.

I had the thought the other night after watching the movie, *Horse Boy* (brilliant film by the way), that I am mentally ill, that I have a mental illness and have had one most of my life and that life maybe would have been and could be a lot easier if I just admitted that. But then I have this fear of being … of being … judged? Locked up? Drugged up? I'm not sure. Yeah, I'm afraid that I'll have my freedom taken away and that my parents will take control of my life and force me to do things the way they think I should do them. It has been quite a wild and crazy ride living inside this mind of mine. It's quite incredible what I've accomplished considering it. It's all perspective, isn't it?

The concept of forgiving oneself really resonates with me today, too. My friend, Rena, talked about it, and it was in the movie *Eat, Pray, Love*. I'm kind of afraid of my parents' visit next week. I don't like being around them when I'm in these places of uncertainty as they like to meddle so much and to try to fix and solve my life. Maybe it's time for a discussion about that. I know that I am special, as is each and every one of us, and each of us is a unique and precious expression of God, of the Divine. Why isn't that enough? It is enough, Shaeah. It has to be enough, anything else is suffering. It's time to put a stop to the unnecessary suffering I cause myself in my own life. Yes, that brings a deeper breath and a smile to my face. Slowly but surely, I am getting it and things are sinking in. I may be a slow learner sometimes, but at least I am a determined one.

I wonder if and who this book will help or inspire? Will it be of benefit to others? Or is it just another one of my delusions? Honey, there I go again … argh!! Okay, another opportunity to practise self-compassion and trust. This is me, this is an expression of me, this is my unique gift … from my heart to yours. It is enough, it is good, it will serve, for that is my intention. So be it and so it is.

August 24

I had a big wake-up call from my body last night. Woke up in the middle of the night with a stomach ache and felt nauseous. Went to the bathroom and in the midst of projecting out both ends, I made a commitment to my body to treat it with more respect. It's time to take full responsibility for my health and well-being. Treat my body like the temple that it is. Love, honour, cherish and respect it. Enough pissing around. So, needless to say, I lost a session today and am missing the first night of ForestFest due to my stupid indulgence. I ate an entire bag of Bamba (an Israeli junk food—actually known to be their national food, they even feed it to babies). It has pretty good ingredients actually, just peanuts and oil, but I think it was eating the whole bag that did me in, plus they may have been off as it does feel like food poisoning. Either way, it's a big clear message to start taking better care of my body. It's also got me thinking about the other areas of my life where I have not been taking full responsibility or, as Donna Martin puts it, response-ability.

Well, let's take a good honest look and see what areas of my life are lacking, not working or, at least, are not to my satisfaction. I guess finances come to mind. I'm not in dire straits or anything, but there is definitely room for improvement. What would taking full responsibility in that area look like? That's the big question; I don't even know how to do it. There are ideas I've had that I haven't taken action on that could potentially bring in more income for me. That would be making my yoga video and meditation CD. I've definitely been stalling on those two projects. Not sure why. Fear, I guess. New territory. What if they fail? What if they suck and no one buys them? I do get people asking me for them. I really do just need to step up and do them. Ok, I will. The completion of this book is a potential income earner. And I've been stalling on this project a lot, too. Getting a master's degree or some further education, but that would mean going more into debt first. Still not sure about that, but interested enough to keep exploring the options. I have been doing some research into online master's degrees. I'm open to the possibility of studying more about psychology and getting a master's in psych.

I was listening to Shimshai in the bath this morning and the lyrics from his song, "Way Within," were perfect to my situation and exactly what I needed to hear:

> We are the temple of the way within, we hold the answer to our deepest questions and when we find the way to living, balance with all that we're given then we begin to find the meaning of this life we're living.

Life keeps guiding me to continue connecting deeper and deeper within.

About fifteen years ago, I went into one of those new age, crystal-type stores on the Sunshine Coast and pulled a piece of paper that the owner had written a little message on. My message said, "You are the love you dream of, the peace you seek, the wholeness you desire. Know this truth and all else will follow."

I remember thinking, "What the hell does that mean?" And I've been on the search to understand that quote ever since. Doubting, questioning, fighting, sometimes kicking and screaming—most of the way. I think I am just starting to understand it. Possibly, not even sure about it. But closer than I've ever been, with still some skepticism and doubt.

August 27

I woke up this morning wondering what it's supposed to feel like to be a woman. A full-grown woman. I still feel like a kid or maybe more like an adolescent at times. I wonder if I come across as being a woman or more like a child? On the weekend, I recognized those patterns of being an adolescent girl looking for attention and wanting to be seen. I guess if I ever get over those patterns I may become a woman? Not sure. Is it possible to ever get over those feelings? My friend was sharing that she had the same feelings and, in her seeking that attention, I felt a little betrayed as she sought it from a man I had told her I was interested in. Perhaps we don't need to get rid of those desires or feelings, but what marks a mature woman is the choice to not act on them. Or is that simply dishonest and inauthentic? No, I believe that there's a choice. One of the things that we do have choice and control over is our actions. How we choose to act and then how we choose to be—our attitude—even though at times it doesn't feel like I have choice in that area. I guess that's another sign of maturity, when one is able to have dominion over their own thoughts, feelings and actions.

September 6

I had a fascinating session with the famous John Preston today. *A local acupuncturist healer.* He covered a lot of territory. From pre-birth to present. Parental influence, heart, mind, body, energy. He touched on things I've been intuiting myself. One, that it would be good to go somewhere warm this winter. He suggested Hawaii or Central America. He agreed that I'm not strong enough to go to India quite yet. He worked on opening my central channels, front and back. He expressed a wish for me to meet a wealthy, sexy man to spend a year or so with, who would pamper and take care of me, so I could just rest and enjoy life. I really like that idea. He also thought it would be good for me to go back to school to get a master's or to become a physician assistant (PA). He said it would help with my confidence and give me a bona fide outlet for the flow of my love and care. He mentioned how our parents are us. My parents are me. They make up who I am, the bricks and mortar, and it's when we realize that and embrace it that we gain all of our chi. Sometimes we have to wait until they die, but we don't have to. He said my life practice is to simply breathe. To just be with my breath as it is, not to try to breathe in any particular way. That I'm to stop trying hard, to let go of doubt and certainty both and to be more in the not knowing. He also wished for me a spiritual master, whatever that means. Soften my eyes, stop looking/seeking outside, settle more into myself and know that the answers are within. There we go again, it keeps coming back to that, to me. He said I might have some intense dreams tonight. He said that my memory issues are related to my compromised adrenals. He joked about getting a t-shirt that says, "Don't ask me, I don't know anything."

As I was walking in the woods afterward, I had the thought that my mission is to not have a mission. He suggested that my life be about having fun, living my joy, which is different from pleasure.

He's definitely feeding into my fantasy. A rich man, a spiritual master, enjoy life, live my joy, have fun, all sounds amazing to me. I told him, "Sign me up!" He was happy to hear that I'd given up on my mission to save the world. I still have some dismantling to do to give that one up fully. That mission lingers but definitely isn't as strong as it's been. I looked up the training for a PA. I would have to go to school in Ontario or Manitoba, and I don't think that's going to happen. I'm leaning more and more toward a master's degree in psychology. Or I guess I could reconsider an education degree.

Life certainly is fascinating. As always, I'm curious to see how it all unfolds. I wonder if the magic of life can be as simple as becoming aware of a possibility and opening up to it, then presto—it can happen. We'll see. I'm so open to a rich, sexy benefactor coming into my life. I have no pride. I'd be happy to surrender to being taken care of for a while. He confirmed my intuitions that I need to rest more, take it easy, have more fun. He said it would be someone who would make me laugh a lot. I'm so sold. Alright, Universe, I put out the call, the classified ad is posted. Wealthy, sexy, fun, loving man to pamper and dote on beautiful, loving, sexy redhead. It would be awesome if the spiritual teacher and rich, sexy lover came in the same package. But I'm not fussy. ;-) Well, we'll see what life has in store. I think it should be a fun and interesting winter. Yippee!!

SEPTEMBER 8

I'm struggling today. Deep fatigue. Feeling lost, confused, disconnected, uninspired. Out of touch. In pain. Sad, tired. I don't know what's wrong, just that I feel that something is wrong. The same old fucking story. Out of sorts. Where has my mojo gone? My joie de vivre? Part of me feels like I need to just leave everything behind and just go on a walkabout. But as I write that it seems like I'd be running away, avoiding. What am I trying to run away from? These feelings of emptiness. Like my life is meaningless. And I feel so ashamed. I can't have anyone know how I really feel. It's embarrassing. I should have it more figured out. I should know better by now. I should have more purpose, more magic, more something, anything. Why am I my own worst enemy? I just want to so escape these feelings. Want to put on a movie, even having thoughts of drinking, of smoking dope. I feel like I need some Divine intervention. But again is that me trying to escape my life as it is? Probably. Avoiding responsibility. But I don't know what to do. I feel pulled in fifty million directions, so then I think, "Well then, I probably need to sit tight, be still and wait. Listen. Allow. Trust." Argh! So frustrating. Where has my magic gone?

SEPTEMBER 11

**It is better to strive in one's own dharma
than to succeed in the dharma of another. Nothing is ever
lost in following one's own dharma. But competition in
another's dharma breeds fear and insecurity.
~ Krishna, *The Bhagavad Gita***

During my walk today, I was contemplating the prospect of creating myself, what that means and what it would look like. If I could truly create myself, what would I create myself as? What would totally tickle my fancy? Someone with a PhD or a master's? Sounds kind of heady and boring. Okay, something more exotic—a dancer or performer of some sort? A dancer like Margie Gillis maybe, not someone with a perfect body and form. More like a free-form performer. Should I apprentice under her? A Cirque du Soleil clown!! Now that excites me. A filmmaker?

So many ideas and possibilities, I got confused and overwhelmed by it all and gave up on the exercise for a while. At some point it struck me, again, it's not about the form or expression, it's about the essence! What essence of being do I want to create myself as? That's easy. Loving, present and grateful were the three things that came right away and then a couple of others: generous, aware. I needed another vowel to be able to make an acronym. I for inspirational. PALGIG. Present, Aware/Accepting, Loving, Generous, Inspirational, Grateful. That is who I am creating myself to be.

I also contemplated the possibility of adding more structure and discipline to my life. Just as an experiment. I thought I'd give it thirty days and see what happens. The new moon is soon, so it's perfect—I'll start then. I'll work out a schedule and stick to it. I was my most clear and inspired during and after that five days of Vipassana where I had a very strict and disciplined schedule and regime. Maybe that's how I do thrive. My sense is it's a balance of the two—structure and flow, of course. The ongoing dance between the opposites.

I had angry resentful thoughts toward John Preston today for feeding my fantasy and disempowering me by suggesting external forces will benefit/save me. A wealthy lover, a spiritual master. Crazy shit. Puts me in that seeking/needing mode. I half wonder if he suggested it in jest to burn out the last vestiges of that part of me that is secretly yearning for that saviour to fix my life and make it all better. *I had concern about keeping this part in about John as it can be interpreted as slander or hurtful, but I felt it was an integral part of my journey of breaking free, so I checked in with John to see if he was okay with it, and this is what he wrote back: "As far as what you have written, I am totally fine with it … What we talk about in session comes from the cloud of information that is around you. Then I tug on bits of it to see how your field moves. A good session is one in which the field moves enough to let the person get freer … I do not release anyone until I know that some of that has happened." I have the utmost respect and love for John and see that he is just representing/ reflecting a dynamic that I am sorting out in myself and that it is not personal to him.*

I wonder if Donna Martin is perhaps the spiritual master and maybe I should go and spend time with her. Life is so strange. Wild, weird and wonderful.

I also keep having thoughts about the book idea: Money, Men and Magic. It keeps haunting me. Perhaps it is my ticket to fortune. If I can create myself as anything, I would love to create myself as wealthy. What the heck. Why not? I'm done with this poverty shit. It's a tiresome game. Done, I say. It'll be fascinating to see how it all unfolds.

SEPTEMBER 13

I wish I had a contraption that captured my thoughts directly. I get the most brilliant ideas while I'm meditating, walking, washing the dishes or bathing and, when I come to write, I'm at a loss. A lot has been happening. Magic, challenge, connection, self. Ocean time, forest time, friend time, solo time, client time. Red dragonfly magic—it landed on my hand three times. *My friend Leslie demonstrated generosity by tipping me $50 and helped me change my acronym from PALGIG to PIGGALA: Present, Inspirational, Generous, Grateful, Accepting, Loving, Adventurous.* PIGGALA's can fly! ;-) Exploring what it means to consciously create myself.

Finding it odd that I'm torn between listening to people's problems all the time and making people laugh. *Seems like a no brainer.* I guess it could be a combo of the two.

Still trying to determine what's mine, what's been inherited, programmed, adopted, implanted. Finding it fascinating that it's so difficult to know what's in my heart, to know how I would choose to live my life if I lived my dream. So many possibilities.

I was reflecting on this book today while I was sitting at the beach. Doubting, questioning, thinking that I'm not sophisticated enough, not profound enough and that people want to read fiction ... blah blah blah. Then I thought, "Well, that's not giving you, the reader, much credit." What if you are deeply yearning for and hungry for raw, real, honest, vulnerable sharing, and you don't even know it or maybe you do. It comes back to trust. Trusting and honouring myself and that which wants to come through me. Leslie gave me the book, *It's Time to Dance* by Tama Kieves. It really is time to live my true joys, loves, passion and dreams. No more excuses, no one to blame. Time to take full responsibility for my own life, my own well-being, my own happiness. Not that I haven't already to some degree, I guess I'm just ready for the next level.

During my meditation, I had the thought that I think I do really have some mental illness of some kind and that it's quite amazing what I've accomplished so far considering. Or maybe the perceived 'mental illness' has been another way to escape responsibility. But I have truly struggled. It's been a battle with my mind to get this far. But luckily, I think I can say that I'm winning. Or who knows? I really don't know anything. I'm intrigued and fascinated to see how it all unfolds. My life, this world, this civilization. I feel like I need to do another big brainstorming session about my life and the way it would look like in my wildest dreams. But not tonight. A project for another time. Now it's time to sleep.

September 18

Existence is waiting for you to flower,
Waiting for you to dance your dance,
Waiting for you to sing your song.
~ Jerru Kabbal

What is my deepest heart's desire? I don't even know anymore. Or maybe I do, and I'm just not willing to admit it, or the desire has been buried under the layers of denial, resistance and fear for so long. There's something going on in here. Inside this aching body is an aching heart. Longing … to be free, to be honoured, to be trusted and listened to. Why don't they teach us this stuff?! I feel angry and sad and confused. So many 'callings.' Which way do I turn?

Okay, let's take some time to explore this. Deep breath, sigh. I close my eyes and delve into the depths of my soul. I see a swirling of colour and movement, long flowing fabrics twirling, dancing. Faces of delight, wonder, awe. I'm terrified. What does this mean? Where does it take me? How do I start? Voices: you're too old, how stupid, what a fantasy, how unrealistic, maybe on the side … on the side of what? I don't want my dream to be plopped on my plate like a side dish.

Dance! What the fuck?! Where, how, with who? What kind? How do I know? Trust, listen, just start. So many questions. Does that mean I have to leave Cortes? Is that how I will make my living? What else do I do if anything? How will I know what that is? A quiet calm voice answers, "It will come, just start." Start how, where, with who? I'm not disciplined and inspired enough to do it on my own. No one here is offering classes. My God, I am so terrified. Why so much fear?! Where does it come from? What am I afraid of? Ridicule, judgment, disappointment. Being wrong, failing, looking stupid.

September 21

Fall equinox—the weather turned cool and grey today as if to honour the day, this change of season. A great time for introspection. *I'm taking Donna Martin's Loving Presence Workshop.* I've been really up against it, yet again. This time with a clearer perspective and understanding of what's happening. By putting my attention on practicing Loving Presence, all that isn't that is rearing its oh-so-lovely, ugly head. I did a yoga practice this morning and tried Donna's approach of just noticing what's happening, did some poses to notice how it felt, then noticed what wanted to happen and was in that exploration for a while.

During it, I had a realization that I don't know how not to try to make something happen. Or, at least, I'm not sure if I know how to let that go. It's so entrenched and ingrained in me to be in control. That brought up a lot of sadness—seeing how hard I'm trying to make something happen all the time. So much unnecessary 'efforting.' A lack of trust in the 'Higher Power' and/or in others. But I also have a lack of trust in myself that I've been getting to see more and more clearly. Not trusting myself is so painful, and it results in so much confusion and inability to move forward. I feel stuck in this perspective that something's wrong, that I need to be fixed, that I'm broken.

Today we practised being in the space of not knowing. I had this amazing feeling of being part of the oceanic waves, the waves of prana. It was both visual and visceral. It's such an amazing shift in consciousness to go from 'there's something wrong' to seeing the gift in every person and situation, including myself and my own experience. Donna mentioned loving oneself and said that in the practice of loving another, we come to love ourselves more. So much learning. Loving Presence is the practice of seeing and even appreciating the gift in each person and each situation. Letting myself be

From My
Heart
To Yours

nourished by the experience. An energy of receiving and allowing evokes an outpouring of positive loving energy, which creates the flow of giving and receiving simultaneously. There's a quality of fluidity, softness, gentleness, spaciousness and grace to this way of being. I like it. I like how it makes me feel, I like what it makes possible. I feel connected, optimistic, grateful and whole.

I had a profound experience during one of the Psoma Yoga sessions. I became present to and shared with the group my feeling of being contained and isolated and my feeling of being stuck in my own shell. We did a process in which the others took over the shell physically and energetically so I could experience what was underneath it. I was able to completely relax and let go, I felt myself soften the hard edges of my being without the need to uphold that shell. I realized how much energy I had been using to keep that shell in place. It felt so good to let go of that efforting. A huge relief. After a while I had this impulse and need to emerge out of the shell, so the others released their envelopment, and I felt myself rise and expand like a butterfly spreading its wings for the first time and being free from the cocoon. It was an incredible feeling. I felt energized, alive, strong, beautiful and free.

SEPTEMBER 22–DECEMBER 15

Wow! Okay, big gap here. I obviously got very distracted. After I emerged from my cocoon, I had a renewed sense of enthusiasm for life. I felt empowered and inspired to create the life I wanted for myself. I made the decision to finally make my dream of living in the tropics for the winter a reality. I did it. I made the decision, made the appropriate arrangements and made it so. Done, "poof like that!", being the powerful and magical being that I am. ;-)

DECEMBER 16
COSTA RICA

**All our dreams can come true,
if we have the courage to pursue them.
~ Walt Disney**

I have arrived! I am in the most exquisitely beautiful place. In the tropics of Costa Rica. Sitting in front of a lotus pond with fuchsia dragonflies, hummingbirds, butterflies, birds of paradise and the most incredible bird songs. Everything is lush green. The ocean kisses the sky on the horizon. Gorgeous structures made of bamboo, wood and artistically sculptured walls. The flower of life, Mayan symbols. This is paradise. For real. A yoga studio overlooks the jungle canopy and the ocean. Feels so incredibly amazing to be here.

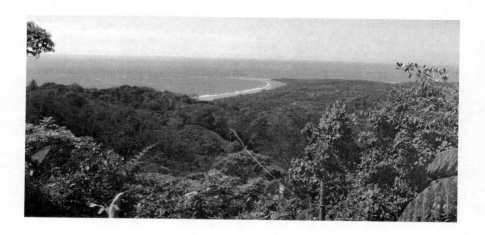

Shaeah Love : **227**

This is my first time writing since I arrived two weeks ago. I have been quite busy getting settled in, finding a place to live, classes, sessions, making connections, socializing. Excuses, excuses. ;-). It's been a powerful time and, at times, challenging. I've been up against my insecurities: doubting, questioning and comparing myself. Mostly in regards to teaching. Heidi and Sofiah (the other yoga teachers here) are amazing and powerful women and teachers. I've been feeling inferior and less than, even though people have been telling me they love my classes. I get fewer students so there's enough proof for my mind. The truth is that they are better teachers in some ways, and that's okay. They've been teaching longer and more frequently than I have. And they also have stronger yoga practices and stronger bodies than I do. I've been working on shifting my attitude to see and receive the inspiration that the other teachers are. It's a great opportunity and impetus for me to grow, deepen, expand and strengthen my practice and teaching. Already I'm feeling stronger and healthier in my body. My mind is getting there. The amazing people who I am surrounded by are helping. I have to keep coming back to gratitude and focussing on how blessed I am. My God, Shaeah! You're living your dream. You're in tropical paradise! I need to own and celebrate that. Stop being so hard on myself. Give myself some time and space to come into my own. I AM LIVING THE DREAM!

Wow, this may well have been one of the most amazing days of my life. An incredible day of magic, epiphanies, adventure, beauty, connection, nourishment, movement, nature, community, empowerment … perfection.

I am here to hold space and offer guidance for your journey home, one of exploration and discovery, one of remembering, opening, trusting, allowing, connecting, honouring, loving and celebrating who you are fully and completely. I am coming into my own Self, freeing myself from held beliefs and limitations. Today I freed myself from the belief that I am less than or inferior to. That's old news based on bullshit. It's not true. I am just as worthy and am available to accept and to receive love and support. I am here to express and share myself, my true beautiful essence freely, fully and unconditionally. I have so much to share and offer. I am here to transmit and model a life of wonder, joy, love, creativity, generosity, beauty, fun, freedom and trust. My life is a canvas, my life is an expression of my art. I am free to express myself creatively in whatever way I choose.

From My
Heart
To Yours

And I choose to express myself with colour, beauty, love, kindness, humour, fun, playfulness, inspiration, magic … I am in paradise. All of my dreams and visions are coming true. Anything in my heart is possible once I believe and allow it to be. And then so much more beyond my expectations and imagination. I feel so blessed.

Our minds can limit us or set us free. It is our choice and that which we cultivate will determine our experience of life and of ourselves. With the willingness to deepen our awareness of Self and the ways we operate, we can attain higher and greater levels of consciousness, freedom, fulfillment, connection and love.

My body is a guide, a map to my soul's calling. Listen to your own tender hearts and follow the call of your own soul. Awaken to your greatest and fullest expression of who you are.

I am surrounded by the songs of the jungle. Frogs, rain, birds, insects, the distant roar of the surf. This place is pure magic, paradise. Faery land. All that I have envisioned possible. So blessed so blessed so blessed. Blessed be!!

DECEMBER 19

I was dealt my own lesson today. The theme of my class this morning was how the mind creates suffering by wanting things to be different than how they are. The practice is to be with and allow what's so. Of course, later that day I found myself resisting and judging my own experience, wanting things and myself to be different. I didn't want to feel sad; instead, I wanted to be somewhere else. With the reflection of a friend, I was able to catch myself and shift into the allowing and being with my experience. I let myself feel the sadness fully and felt an exquisite sense of release and cleansing from letting my tears flow. It's okay to be sad; in fact, when I don't resist the feeling, it feels really good. Liberating, in fact. Healing. A softening naturally began to happen as the edges of my resistance dissolved. I now feel more at peace and simply, sweetly okay. I meditated shortly after this process and release, to give myself time to be with myself in stillness and silence. As I began meditating, I was bombarded by unwanted sounds, the loud rev of a motorcycle, pounding of nails, beeping of horns, barking of dogs. It was so perfectly not the environment 'conducive' to a peaceful meditation that I began to laugh and cry at the same time at the absurdity and humour of the situation. The perfect opportunity to practise once again—accepting and allowing the situation to be what it is. My reactivity subsided and, with it, the sounds. I was able to sink into a deep and fulfilling meditation.

Now I find myself even more at ease and at peace within myself. My awareness has expanded to include more of my environment. I equally hear the songs of the birds and feel the soft breeze on my skin. I believe that sadness and any emotion is the language of my soul speaking to me. Calling me to awaken and remember why I am here. I feel a call to be of greater service. I feel called to contribute to the community in some way whereas before I was feeling separate and judgmental. Not wanting to be here. Now I feel compelled to

From My
Heart
To Yours

reach out and connect. We are such fascinating creatures. At least I am to myself. Both intriguing and infuriating. The great paradox of life.

DECEMBER 20

Last night I had an angel reading and healing with an incredibly beautiful, lovely new soul sister, Danielle. It was so powerful and perfect. The reading/channeling was about self-love, purity of heart and being supported. The reading encouraged me to pursue counselling, to focus on my health, to connect with nature, passion and gentleness. She/they said I am done with my karmic debt, and they will help me clear out any lingering fear or blocks to the flow of my love and light. They said to focus on my steps toward being a counsellor, and they will light the way. I am on the path. I'm doing good work, keep it up. Trust, stop worrying, ask and receive their guidance and support. She also said to pay attention to my dreams. So last night I set the intention to be aware of my dreams and to learn from them. I woke up from an intense dream about fighting for my life, being on the defense and running away from people who were trying to kill me and each other. At one point, I took a hostage so no one would shoot me. At the end, I managed to run away into a building, found a pair of scissors and a video camera and cornered myself into the back of a room. Another woman found me who also had scissors. When we were face to face, scissors pointed at each other, I told her I wouldn't hurt her if she wouldn't hurt me. I think she walked away, and that's when I woke up. When I meditated on the meaning or message of the dream, I got that I and many others are still living in fight-or-flight survival mode. I am focussed on my survival, my needs, my interests. Focussed on staying alive and on what's in it for me. Protection. Guarded. Separate.

It's time to shift this attitude of survival to one of cooperation, collaboration, trust and compassion. When I asked how to shift out of the defensive/aggressive mode, I received the message "to surrender. Let go of my own agenda and strategies for survival. Focus on helping others, focus on sharing and contributing and loving. Soften the hard edges of protection and resistance that keep me separate and alone." I think that's why I felt sad yesterday. I could feel my separateness as I walked around town; I was judging, being on guard, feeling out of place, focussing on what I wanted to get instead of what I have to give. I'm so done with this mode of being. It feels shitty and doesn't serve anyone including myself.

I don't want to do life on my own anymore. Life is meant to be shared, co-created and celebrated with others. I'm so excited about this shift. It's been a long time coming. I have been aware of and have felt the entrapment of this way of being, but I didn't know how to get out of it, it's been so ingrained. Now I feel that with the help of the angels and my soul sisters and brothers, it is possible. It is time.

A small voice questions whether it's too idealistic, but I don't care. It's too painful to live any other way. It's worth the risk of 'getting hurt' or 'being disappointed.' The only way this shift will happen is if we just start and do our best to live from a place of love rather than fear, one step at a time, and if we continue to be gentle with ourselves, forgive ourselves when we falter and begin again. A wise teacher once said, "A true master is not one who has perfected a way of doing something, a true master is one who gets up after every time she stumbles or falls. It is the courage, the commitment, the willingness to continue on the path no matter what, in the face of any challenge or seeming failure." Master, student—it's all the same to me. What matters is continuing to live my life with as much heart, gratitude and generosity as possible. And so the shift happens … one thought, word or action at a time.

My vision for what's possible. The world I am choosing to co-create looks like this:

- Clean air, clean water, clean earth—adequate nourishment for all—body, mind, heart & spirit

- Kindness towards all beings

- Love, compassion, acceptance, support, care, respect, honour

- Co-creation, celebration

- Generosity, sharing, giving, expressing generously

- Freedom of expression without harm

- Appreciation and gratitude

- Connection, community, togetherness

- Devotion—in service and contributing to the benefit of others

- Creativity, life as art

- Play, humour, joy

- Divine inspiration

- Freedom & liberation

- Curiosity, wonder, awe & magic

- Willingness & cooperation

- Understanding & communication—authenticity & honesty

- Peace—non-violence

From My
Heart
To Yours

DECEMBER 22

Well, the world didn't come to an end, as some predicted it might. Maybe, hopefully, some aspects ended/died. We can only hope. We had an amazing celebration last night. So beautiful. We shared delicious food, prayer, ceremony, connection and dance. A lot of joy was created and shared. As Dawn (another new soul sister) said, "That's one of the most healing things we can do, to feel and emanate joy."

Yes, my heart is full and happy with a remnant of sadness. Sad from not being with family and other friends. Sad because there still is so much suffering on the planet. Not sure that will ever change. But at least I'm not suffering as much.

December 23

It is in the act of loving and accepting every aspect of who I am that I become whole, I naturally attract all that I desire.
~ Shaeah Love

I'm taking a day of rest! No looking at the clock, just listening to my body and giving it what it needs and wants. Right now it wants rest. I'm feeling called to write. Not sure what about, feeling a little self-doubting these days, but I just know that the commitment to and the practice of writing is what's important. It's building trust in myself. Building confidence that I have something worthwhile to say. Or not. It doesn't really matter. It's the act of honouring myself that matters.

I'm pretty much loving my life. Yeah, very much. I'm living in paradise, near a river and the ocean. Banana and papaya trees are practically at arm's reach from my house. Last night, stars and fireflies twinkled my path home. I'm getting in great shape. Walking, swimming, doing Heidi's kick-ass yoga class. She's inspiring. Hosting events, teaching classes, giving awesome sessions. Eating really well. Softening the self-critic and inner judge Feeling more at ease in myself. Feeling really grateful and blessed to be where I am. Mostly thrilled about the people I'm connecting with. Love my home. I'm feeling the most 'in integrity' than I ever have. Heidi's class was about integrity yesterday. I love how she weaves her theme in through the whole class. Something I aspire to. I've made huge progress since I've been here. I love that I'm getting stronger and buffer. I can notice more ease in my sessions due to my increased core strength. I'm feeling that I want to offer courses on it: core strength and body awareness for bodyworkers.

I really love and appreciate the connection to the angels. I feel like I'm not alone anymore. Wow, I'm so addicted to time. I'm dying to know what time it is. It feels so good to be lazing around in bed, writing and daydreaming. I'm feeling the need to connect with someone. An urge to get on Facebook or send an email. So many ways I distract myself. I also noticed today that I love bookkeeping. I love keeping track of my money and spending. It's fun. I wonder if I will ever be rich. I'm rich in so many ways, but I wonder if I'll ever shift my money dynamics. I think so. It's just a matter of time. I'm a manifester after all. I keep feeling called to that book: Money, Men and Magic. I could just start and see what happens. I wonder if I'll ever finish this one. It's up to me. Oh, big sigh. So happy, content, fulfilled, grateful. Yep, feeling good. Yay me!

DECEMBER 28

Big sigh. I've been struggling a bit. With that whole self-love thang. The critic and judge running rampant about my yoga classes and my teaching style. Comparing myself to others, feeling uninspired, not enjoying teaching yoga. It sucks. I'm wondering why, am curious. Which of course is a good thing. One thing in my favour. During my sunrise beach walk this morning, I asked myself, "What's out? What do I need to do differently?" And what came is that I need to do my own personal practice more regularly. I've barely been doing any of my own personal practice. Just been teaching and going to classes. I need to reconnect with why I love yoga for myself and why I chose to teach it in the first place. Why did I? I remember that feeling of coming home to myself. A calming down. Things became less of a problem. I felt more at ease within myself and with life. I felt stronger and healthier. My body began to relax and open up more. My mind became quieter, and I became more present. The pain in my body became manageable and bearable. I actually would feel good in my body.

January 6

My first entry of the new year. A lot has been happening, shifting, opening. I had a huge revelation this morning in a Psoma Yoga session with my dear friend, Erin, over Skype. Since I've come to Costa Rica, I've been struggling with intense self-judgment, criticism and even self-loathing. So much so that I've been considering to quit teaching yoga. I haven't been enjoying teaching classes because all the way through the class I am judging myself as a shitty teacher and projecting that the students are judging me too, not enjoying themselves and are thinking that I suck. It's been brutal. When I got quiet and asked myself what to do about this and how to shift this, I was guided to reconnect with the reason I started teaching and to amp up my own personal practice. Which I haven't really done yet. Something has been getting in the way, my patterns of self-sabotage in full gear.

Anyway, the point is that this morning while investigating these feelings of sadness and heaviness from this lack of self-love, I discovered that it's the form of masculine love I know from both of my father figures. Rather than feeling loved, supported and protected, I felt judged, attacked and threatened. So this is how I've come to know how to express and receive masculine love. When I got this realization, I decided that I don't want to operate in this way anymore but to instead focus on being loving, supportive and protective to myself and be open to receiving that from others. Erin affirmed that now that this has been brought to my consciousness, I can catch it and make new choices. I felt an opening and release of knotting and tension in my jaw and stomach. By the end of the session I felt clear, open, happy and a flow of love in my body, mind and energy. I love Psoma Yoga. It's so simple and powerful. I must keep remembering and tapping into it. I'm glad that I followed my pull to reach out to Erin and Don *(my Psoma Yoga cohorts)*. We are going to stay in contact regularly. This is really important. I must remember and practise this level of awareness and this way of being that is pure Loving Presence.

My intention for this year is to ever expand my capacity to love and receive love. LOVE FLOW!

JANUARY 14

Do you also have an ungrateful bitch living inside of you? Isn't she annoying? No matter how great things are, she's gotta find something that is shitty or not to her 'standards.'

JANUARY 16

I invite you to go to the most still place you have ever been. Deep inside.

Expanding awareness to include your whole experience. Unite all aspects of who you are with your awareness and your breath.

I had a bunch of epiphanies today …

I must see the God in you and in everyone to truly be free.

Be all of it and none of it at the same time. That which is connected to it all and free from all of it. Not attached yet completely engrossed. Absorbed even. Alignment, stillness, awareness, breath, expanding and contracting. All and none all at once.

JANUARY 28

Our deepest fear is not that we are inadequate. Our deepest fear is that we are powerful beyond measure. It is our light, not our darkness that most frightens us. We ask ourselves, Who am I to be brilliant, gorgeous, talented, fabulous? Actually, who are you not to be? You are a child of God. Your playing small does not serve the world. There is nothing enlightened about shrinking so that other people won't feel insecure around you. We are all meant to shine, as children do. We were born to make manifest the glory of God that is within us. It's not just in some of us; it's in everyone. And as we let our own light shine, we unconsciously give other people permission to do the same. As we are liberated from our own fear, our presence automatically liberates others.
~ Marianne Williamson, *A Return To Love*

I've been stuck in a funk. Same familiar cycle of self-limitation, deprivation, and a toned-down, less-than-full-life ME. Feeling sorry for myself, needing to put others down to feel good about myself. Insecure and self-punishing. I've been avoiding things that I want to do or to achieve. I think I'm doing my best to love myself and doing the best I can do, and yet I know I am capable of more. And then I think of Pema Chodron's quote that says something like even the desire to change is a slight act of violence to oneself. What's fascinating is that in the Google search for the exact words of that quote I found a website that read, "Stop trying to accept yourself" and that trying to accept yourself is stupid or something. I'm not quite getting it yet. But I love that I found a site espousing the exact opposite message and, therefore, perspective.

I've been thinking a lot lately about fluidity and the ability to flow between various perspectives and points of view. It's hard to see me act through my ego filter. As always, I'm feeling caught between two worlds, wondering if I'm truly crazy, wishing I was living more boldly, expressing myself more fully and freely. Trying my best but knowing there's so much more. Afraid to break out, not sure of what? Of being seen? Failing? There's no failing in trying.

I feel a strong pull to dance more and to get more outrageous, theatrical, courageous, bold and daring. To step into a different way of being. I've done insecure, unsure, self-conscious a lot—I have got it down. Time to try something new. Bold, courageous, confident, successful, daring, beautiful, shining. Why not? What do I have to lose? I've been inspired by the show *Glee* and by my little sister winning Miss Teen Alberta-World. She is an amazing young woman. Living boldly, pursuing her dreams. She's so sure of herself and she's only 17! We don't connect often, but when we're together, pure love is present. One of my favourite things is to cuddle with her on the couch while watching TV. My brother and sister are from my dad's second marriage and are young enough to be own children. We have a very special bond.

My brother and I had the most amazing talk the other night. The best connecting ever. I've been yearning for this day for a long time. Sometimes you gotta let something go before it can come to you. He wanted to be mentioned in this book, so now he is. I love him so.

I'm feeling out of integrity in certain areas of my life. Relationship, self-care, life purpose. Time to get back in the groove. My groove, the Shaeah groove. Be proud of who I am, own it, claim my life and live it fully.

Oh, interesting, I just found the quote:

Even the desire to change
is a subtle form of violence toward oneself.
~ Pema Chodron

I was pretty close. As always, a constant dance between two opposing energies, the paradox of life. Gotta love it.

JANUARY 30

Hmmm … struggling a bit. Not sure what to do, what to say. Feeling a bit lost. Sad, confused. A little out. Not quite in integrity but not sure how to get there. I'm feeling stuck between that place of wanting to be happy with and accept who I am and of desiring to be different, better, stronger, healthier. Is it truly bad to want to be better? To want to change? Isn't that a natural part of who we are? We are destined to change and evolve. It's our nature so why not want to influence how and what we change into? It comes down to the conundrum of will versus surrender again.

I'm in total avoidance. I notice all of my tactics for avoiding are in full force. Eating, Facebooking, feeling the pull to watch videos. Argh! What am I avoiding?

I've also been taking care of some things that I've been putting off, which feels good. Getting in integrity with my communications. Completing communication cycles.

I'm looking for something. Some validation, some inspiration. I feel my Spirit is wanting something from me, trying to tell me something, guiding me toward something, but I'm not sure what. I'm not sure if it's my ego or my heart that's being pulled toward being … *Hmmm … what could I have possibly been going to say? What interrupted me? A-ha, the mystery of it all. ;-)*

From My
Heart
To Yours

FEBRUARY 17

It's just over a year now since I started writing this. I've had mixed thoughts and feelings about it as always. Mixture of failure, hope, excitement, despair, frustration, criticism, judgment, possibility, curiosity, but what has been missing most is inspiration. Or maybe simply, it's just time that has been missing. I've been busy. And I haven't made time for writing. It hasn't been a priority. Today is the first time in a while I've had any spark of inspiration to write so I decided to 'carpe diem.'

I caught myself starting to make other plans, excuses and luckily I nipped them in the 'butt,' and here I am. Finally. So much to say, so much I could say. That's also part of the challenge, I often don't know where I would start. But that's the point, to not know and to just simply start. (A–ha, full circle! ;-) I pause, close my eyes, take a few conscious breaths, listen to the sound of the jungle and the fan, feel the cool breeze, smell the sweet air and sigh. Here I am. Connect in, tap into what it is I really want to say. I feel so much. Such an array and mix of emotions, feelings, sensations, thoughts. A deep breath, ahh, feels so good. I want to talk about love. I just spent two weeks with my mom, who loves me unconditionally. And I have been on the receiving end of loving attention from a dear man.

Argh, having trouble writing, so jumbled in my mind. Not sure what to say first, how ... It was all so clear just a while ago when I had the first inspiration to write. So much choice. Choice in how we are, in how we choose to act, in what we choose to say, in how we choose to be. And it all comes down to how much love we're willing to put into it all, doesn't it?

Oh yeah, I was having this revelation earlier about all of these people that love me and that I haven't been able to understand why. What is it they see or feel that makes them love me so much? And why can't I feel it, know it or see it? Why can't I love myself as others can and do? Maybe that's not my job, it's not up to me. It's up to me to love others and their job to love me? Yes, that's a question mark, there's uncertainty there. I feel I can and want to be more generous with my love. I feel I hold back. I see where and how I hold back, and it hurts and frustrates me that I do. I wish I could just let my love flow fully and freely without concern or consideration of any kind. Just as God does. That's what I aspire to. Now this is the shit, this is getting real. That is my purpose in life. To love as God loves. Wow! I just got my purpose in life! In a more real way than ever before. It resonates more as truth than ever. I'm getting there. I feel my trust and faith deepening. In myself, in life and in others.

I have no idea what it looks like or exactly how I'm supposed to love as God loves. I don't need to know. All I need is the intention and willingness and to allow the spontaneous expression of Divine Love and Energy to flow through me—as me—for the mutual benefit of others and myself. "I offer myself as a clear and open vessel for Divine Love, Divine Light, Divine Energy and Divine Truth to flow through me, as me for the greatest good of all." How amazing is that?! ;-)

And the journey continues …

I bowed my head to God,
And God took all of me,
Every imperfection,
God took all of me,
And every day,
God lives and breathes through me…
~Snatam Kaur

P.S.

**The future belongs to those who believe
in the beauty of their dreams.
~ Eleanor Roosevelt**

Dreams do come true! I *made* mine come true. Much of the healing I experienced on this journey was sourced in being true to myself and in honouring my visions for what's possible. I wrote and am publishing this book—one of my greatest accomplishments to date—and that feels amazing! It's wild to look back to where I've been and where I am today.

For some unknown reason I stopped writing after that last entry in February. I'm guessing it's because I had less than two months left in Costa Rica and I became engrossed with all the activities and making the most of my time while I was there. When I returned to Canada I realized that it was a great place to finish. But I'd like to fill you in on what has happened since then.

I really came into myself and gained greater clarity, power and freedom from the profound shifts and transformation I experienced during my remaining time in Costa Rica. I identified and released a shell of shyness that was keeping me contained and feeling separate. I attended the festival, Envision, where I was able to express myself and connect with others in a freer, more open and deeper way than ever before.

I read the book, *The Shack*, by W. M. Paul Young and was affirmed that we all have God in us and hence, the ability to touch and affect people in powerful, profound and healing ways. Something I had suspected but hadn't fully embraced or owned. Once I did, my sessions went off the scale. My clients experienced spontaneous healings; after one session, the client said the pain that she had had in her back for years was gone. Another client said he could actually feel the healing happening.

Around that time, by request, I decided to offer a Lomi Lomi training. I became clear that I had a responsibility to pass on the knowledge I had and to help others awaken to their God-given ability to touch people in profound ways. Once I committed to offering the training, it all came together beautifully and filled up with an amazing group of individuals. We had the most exquisite experience of connecting, sharing and healing. I realized that giving Lomi Lomi trainings is an ideal way to share and offer all of my gifts and passions: meditation, movement, bodywork, Loving Presence, prayer, magic, connection, community and celebration.

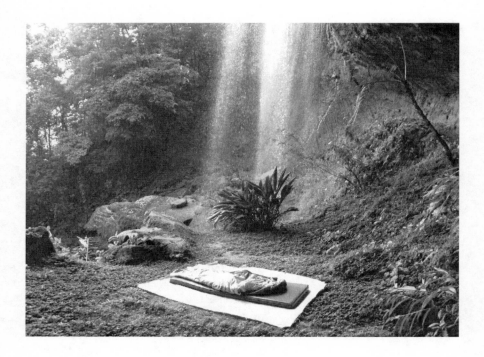

At one point I was called to visit some waterfall caves, Diamante Verde. It was there that I discovered the heart and soul of Costa Rica and Pacha Mama. I sat and meditated right beside the water-fall for hours and experienced a direct connection to Source and to

From My
Heart
To Yours

my inner knowing. I became crystal clear that I needed to publish this book because it is an essential step in my evolution and in me emerging more fully as I am.

I returned to Canada renewed in spirit, strengthened in body, steadfast in mind and expanded in heart. Theda and I co-produced a yoga CD, *Crystal Bowl Yoga Journey*, that has been met with enthusiasm and rave reviews. Once we made the decision to produce the CD, it happened with ease and grace. I decided to self-publish this book. I was inspired by others I knew who had done it and recommended self-publishing as the way to go. The process has been empowering and enlightening. My friend, Theda inspired and supported me to run an Indiegogo campaign to raise the money to publish this book. It was a powerful learning experience and I was blown away by all the generous support I received from my family, friends and greater community.

My relationships have been deepening on all levels. Especially with my immediate family. Despite all of the challenges we've faced and the differences we have, there is deep love and respect between us that continues to grow and deepen. My parents (all three of them) have been an incredible source of support and love. I adore each of them and feel so incredibly blessed to know them and have them in my life.

My dream of true love did come to be. This past summer I met and fell in love with an amazing man, who I truly experience as 'my match made in heaven.' We met at our friends' wedding. How romantic is that?! Our level of connecting and relating is deep, honest, respectful, playful, loving and fulfilling. We are both strong in who we are and are fully devoted to each other in ways that enhance and enrich our lives immensely. The quality of our connection is a testament to the work that I have done to cultivate the ability to love myself as I am and others as they are. I decided not to have children for various reasons and I'm at peace with that decision. I have chosen to be of service and to channel my creative life force in different ways.

I am living my purpose. I am here to love, live and create as fully, freely and generously as possible. I am here to be as beautiful as I can—just as I am. With scars, wrinkles, stretch marks, blemishes, grey hairs, flab and all. I am here to fully love, embrace and express my unique and glorious self as I AM! I am available to serve you in whichever way you need as best as I can, to enhance your life in whatever way possible. I allow Spirit/Divine Essence/Love to flow through me to you.

There's nothing wrong with me, with you or with anything. Nothing to fix. Just the presence of other possibilities to be explored and discovered. We can choose to stay in the same experience as long as we want or, whenever we are ready and willing, we can let go and choose a new and/or different experience. No worse or better. This is freedom. This is liberation.

I continually choose the path of love. My life has become more about being of service and sharing my love more freely and fully. My Beloved jokes that I 'work for big G.' It's true. I believe we all do in our own unique way of being in service. ;-) I am being called to step up more as a leader. To me this means to live and model the life and the way of being that I see possible. This doesn't mean I'm going to run for office or anything, although I am greatly inspired by Marianne Williamson, who recently declared that she is running for congress. I admire that she is taking this stand and that, as she has stated, she is "taking the transformational principles to which I have dedicated myself for the last thirty years into another area where they are sorely needed." She went on to say:

> While a new paradigm, holistic, relational perspective now saturates many areas of our society—from education to business to medicine to spirituality—our politics seem to be outside its reach. And we cannot afford to turn away from politics. We might not touch it, but it certainly touches us. And the increasingly calcified thought forms that dominate U.S. politics today—based more on the past than on the present, more on fear than on love and more on economic than humanitarian values—threaten to sabotage our collective good and undermine our democracy.

I have faith in humanity. Things are changing. We are waking up. We all have our unique role to play in this wild and wacky unfolding of life. I believe that our ongoing practice as responsible conscious beings is to do whatever we can to master our minds, which are connected to our hearts and hence directly affects our ability and capacity to love. It's essential that we continue to be honest with ourselves and with each other as best we can. It is up to us to consciously cultivate ourselves as that which we seek. As the great Gandhi once said:

Be the change that you wish to see in the world.

Personally, I see a new paradigm, a collective of world leaders. We take a stand for world peace, justice, equality and food and clean water for all. We model and teach the values of honesty, respect, care, honour and love. You could be a part of this collective if you so choose. Maybe you already are. Or maybe you have your own creative project to birth. Or perhaps you have your own hero's journey to experience. And most certainly you have your own mystery to unfold. Just remember that flying solo is optional. ;-)

Individually or together we can and will continue to create the world we imagine possible. The most important thing is to be true to yourself and if you don't know what that means then do whatever you can to find out. Let's keep transforming and evolving. It's our destiny. Maybe. Gotta love the Mystery. ;-) LOL!

Our nation, like an individual, is as sick as its secrets—as unhealed as its unlooked at places ... and on its way to transformation to the extent that it's willing to take a good look at itself and change course where needed.
~ Marianne Williamson

EPILOGUE

I'm getting caught up on the seeming finality of this epilogue. Feeling pressure to be profound, meaningful, awe-inspiring, earth-shattering, touching, moving and enlightenting. Wanting desperately to leave you with the most truth imbued, lasting impression possible. I've come to realize that this is mission impossible. First of all, how can anyone perform under such pressure?! And yet this is the way a lot of us try to live our lives. No wonder stress one of is the leading causes of illness. Second, I find it impossible to capture exactly what to say since each day or even each moment brings a new experience that changes my perspective on life. I have this feeling as though I'm playing with mercury, that elusive nature, constantly slipping away from my fingertips. What I am left with is the quote, "The only thing constant is change." Life is too fluid for me to espouse anything that captures absolute truth. So all I can truly share is my experience and what's happening for me in this moment, and that could very well change in the next. That's one of the marvels of life.

This morning while I was meditating in the Notre Dame de Paris seeking clarity from the jumble of thoughts and ideas and hoping to receive inspiration for this epilogue, I realized it's quite simple really. It's in the title of this book: *From My Heart To Yours*. Thus, I come back to my heart, feel out to yours and trust and allow what comes.

From the infinite depth of my heart, "Thank you". Thank you for taking your precious time to read and receive my offering. Thank you for letting me in to your world and into your heart for a while and maybe having an impact on you in some way. Thank you for your energy and support. Thank you for being on this wild and wonder-filled journey with me. I really couldn't have done it without you. Thank you and bless you on your journey and however you choose to live it.

I want you to know that you are not alone. No matter how difficult life seems to get or how much pain or despair you feel, others can relate and will understand your experience. I want to provide the hope and understanding that I wish I had had at those darkest moments I know life's not easy at times; in fact, it can seem downright brutal. I want you to know that if I can overcome, so can you. Even though we are ultimately alone, at the same time, we are all in this together. We each have our unique journey to experience, and yet we all share something in common—the wonders of the human experience and all the joy and pain that comes with it.

For whatever reason, I have struggled with a lot of challenges and suffering, mostly internal. Over the years, I have faced and overcome a lot of inner demons. I have experienced the lowest of the lows, the highest of the highs and many things in between. (I was going to say "everything in between," but that wouldn't be true because there's still so much more to experience). ;-) I realize that the rigidity of my mind in the form of judgments, resistances and preferences are what create most of my suffering. I do my best to stay open as much as I can. When I recognize that I am contracting or judging, I fess up and do my best to release whatever I am holding on to. I do my best to accept all with curiousity and gratitude, this is my pilgrimage of love. I am human, I do falter and each time I do what I can to correct and continue.

I know I'm a good person AND at times I can be critical. I believe in miracles AND at times I have a highly skeptical mind. Sometimes I feel incredibly brilliant and inspired AND at times I feel so lost and even crazy. I strive to make a difference AND sometimes I wish I could disappear. I fantasize that this book will become a best-seller AND I cringe at the thought of the pressure and responsibility of fame. I have big dreams and desires AND ultimately I wish to live a simple life. I am who I am AND I have this miraculous capacity to ever expand and evolve. Amazingly enough one does not negate the other. We have the capacity to hold it all. This is the ongoing dance with the paradox of life. The marvelous messy middle. It's not about one or the other but about embracing the fluctuating fluid nature of our being. We are about 60% water afterall. ;-)

Isn't life fascinating? Don't people constantly astound you? I continue to surprise myself.

By the way, don't believe a word I say. I'm serious. Same goes for anything anyone else tells you including the things your own mind tells you. ;-) I need to say this to set us both free. It's not because what I've told you isn't true. It's because what I've shared with you is MY experience in the moment and was exactly what needed to happen for ME. YOU can discover YOUR own truth and experience YOUR own unique unfolding. Your life is completely unique, and it's important to honour that. I guarantee you that life won't turn out like you expect it to nor like anyone else says it's supposed to be. The wonder of life is that you get to discover it for yourself.

You are welcome to use any of the tools I have shared, but just know that they may not necessarily be the tools that will serve you. My purpose in sharing them was to demonstrate to you that various modes of support can help us get through challenging times or help us to really appreciate the blessings that come our way. It is key to trust that support is there when you need it or, if it isn't, to know that you have the option to seek it out and find it if you want. My experience is that life always brings me what I need and nothing more than I can handle. The more I trust in myself and in the natural unfolding of life, the more enjoyable and richer life becomes.

Trust and surrender. Love, acceptance and gratitude. Life keeps guiding me back to love. When I pair everything else away, I always come back to the essence of being love. Love love love. Love myself as I am, love others as they are, love life as it is. Seemingly so simple, yet incredulously challenging at times. But there's no denying it, love truly does heal; the balm that soothes all wounds. The great news is we all have the ability to love and be loved. And love is the force that unites us all.

May the force be with you…

Where there is love there is life.
~ Mahatma Ghandi

LOVE TO LIVE TO LOVE

**May all beings be happy. May all beings
be peaceful. May all beings be free.**

SO BE IT AND SO IT IS

It happens all the time in heaven,
And some day

It will begin to happen
Again on earth–

That men and women who are married,
And men and men who are
Lovers,

And women and women
Who give each other
Light,

Often will get down on their knees

And while so tenderly
Holding their lover's hand,

With tears in their eyes,
Will sincerely speak, saying,

"My dear,
How can I be more loving to you;

How can I be more
Kind?"

~Hafiz

NOTES

1. Vipassana Meditation, www.dhamma.org

2. Patricia Ryan Madson, www.stanford.edu/~patryan

3. Barefoot Dragonfly, www.thebarefootdragonfly.com/mooncircle.htm

4. Lawrence Noyes, www.lawrencenoyes.com/html/clearing___consulting.html

5. Lazaris. The Sacred Journey; You and Your Higher Self. Appendix Reference Guides Part III, www.lazaris.com

6. Susan Barber, www.spiritofmaat.com/archive/jun3/prns/lazaris.htm

7. Abraham Hicks, Ask and It Is Given, p. 114.

8. Kripalu, www.kripalu.org

9. Okra, www.okracharlotte.com/yoga/ashtanga/

10. Gregor Maehale, Ashtanga Yoga, p. 136.

11. Ian Mackenzie & Velcrow Ripper, Occupy Wall St.—The Revolution of Love with Charles Eisenstein, www.youtube.com/watch?v=BRtc-k6dhgs

12. Long Island Center for Yoga, www.longislandyoga.com/yoga-nidra.html

13. Nauli, www.nauli.org

14. WebMD, www.webmd.com

15. Richard Bock, www.quantumlightbreath.com

16. Graham Wright, Government Explained, based on a talk by Larken Rose www.youtube.com/watch?v=EUS1m5MSt9k

17. Thanissaro Bhikkhu, www.accesstoinsight.org/lib/authors/thanissaro/affirming.html

18. Stephen Cope, Yoga and the Quest for the True Self, p. 138.

19. Art of Living Foundation, www.artofliving.org/yoga-breathing-techniques/alternate-nostril-breathing-nadi-shodhan

20. Begin Within, www.beginwithin.org/freeing-yourself-with-hooponopono/

21. Claudia Yoga, www.earthyogi.blogspot.ca/2011/03/10-things-to-know-about-pratyahara.html

Resources

Personal/Professional/Spiritual Growth

www.alohaloveheals.com (Lomi Lomi Trainings & Sessions)

www.amrityoga.org (Yoga Nidra CD's & Trainings)

www.anjalihill.com (Training For A Better Life)

www.dhamma.org (Vipassana Meditation)

www.donnamartin.net (Psoma Yoga & Hakomi Trainings)

www.hollyhock.ca (Canada's Lifelong Learning Centre; Conferences, Trainings, Workshops, Retreats)

www.kennedylifesolutions.com/ (Enlightenment Intensives & Coaching)

www.kripalu.org/ (Center for Yoga & Health)

www.lawrencenoyes.com (Enlightenment Intensive Trainings, Clearing Trainings and Sadhana Retreats)

www.landmarkworldwide.com (International Personal and Professional Growth, Training and Development Company) www.lazaris.com (A remarkable body of tools, techniques, processes, and pathways for our Spiritual Journey to God/Goddess/All That Is)

www.members.shaw.ca/murei/ (Enlightenment Intensives)

www.paradoxacademy.com (Dyad School for Yoga, Meditation, and Self-Realization Therapy)

www.quantumlightbreath.com (QLB CD & Info)

www.shamanicbodywork.com (Lomi Lomi Trainings & Sessions)

www.warriorsage.com (Ignite Passion, Live Freedom & Embody Love – Trainings & Workshops by Satyen & Suzanne Raja)

Inspiration

www.abraham-hicks.com (Inspirational Words & Workshops)

www.brainyquote.com/ (Great Source for Inspirational Quotes)

www.dalailama.com (Bodhisattva of Compassion)

www.margiegillis.org (Margie Gillis Dance Foundation)

www.mariannewilliamson.com (Internationally Acclaimed Spiritual Author and Lecturer)

www.planetsark.com (Your Home for Dreaming, Daring & Doing)

www.occupylove.org (A Film by Velcrow Ripper)

www.rickhanson.net (Resources for Happiness, Love & Wisdom)

www.thedaphoenix.com (Voice of an Angel; CD's & Events)

Goods & Services

www.britanniabodyworks.com (Calgary Multidisciplinary Health Clinic)

www.costaricaretreatyoga.com/ (Selva Armonia; Re-treat & Eco-lodge dedicated to your highest good)

www.embraceyourdeath.com/ (Stephen Garrett Coaching & Support for facing death)

www.erosha.com (Somatic Sexual Education, Coaching & Healing)

www.halfmoonhaven.com/ (Sunshine Coast Beachfront Retreat & Spa)

www.ianmack.com (Crowdfunding & Filmmaker Extraordinaire)

www.lucentedits.com (Personal Editing Service for the Academic, Business and Non-fiction Writer)

www.majie.ca (My Beloved's Beautiful Art)

www.mulberryland.com (Nico & Naomi teWinkel's Amazing Offerings)

www.ruthozeki.com (Ozekiland; Books)

www.sacred-economics.com (Book by Charles Eisenstein; Money, gift & society in the age of transition)

www.shaeahlove.com (I offer you my love in all it's many expressions)

SHAEAH LOVE FIALKOW

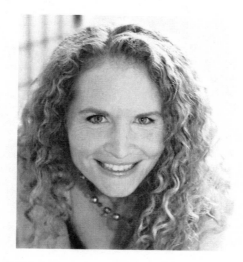

SHAEAH is dedicated to ever awakening, opening, connecting to, living and sharing her deepest heart's truth and calling. Her Love is often expressed as a yoga teacher, transformational life coach, workshop facilitator, bodyworker, radio show host, performer, artist, lover, daughter, sister and friend, and now inspirational author. She lives on the west coast of beautiful British Columbia with her Beloved and their very playful cat. www.shaeahlove.com